QUALITY OF HEALTH CARE FOR OLDER PEOPLE IN AMERICA

A Review of Nursing Studies

Norma M. Lang, Ph.D., R.N., F.A.A.N.
Janet M. Kraegel, Ph.D., R.N.
Marilyn J. Rantz, M.S.N., R.N.
Janet Wessel Krejci, M.S., R.N.

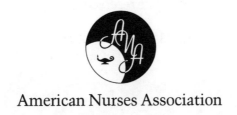

American Nurses Association

Norma M. Lang, Ph.D., R.N., F.A.A.N., is Dean and Professor of the University of Wisconsin-Milwaukee School of Nursing. She is president of the American Nurses Foundation, a member of the Institute of Medicine, and a member of the board of the American Medical Peer Review Association. She was recently appointed as a member of the national advisory board of the Agency for Health Care Policy and Research, advising on quality of health care issues.

Janet M. Kraegel, Ph.D., R.N., most recently was appointed as Associate Chief of Nursing Service for Research at Clement Zablocki Veterans Administration Medical Center in Milwaukee. She has written several books on nursing administration, including *Patient Care Systems: Strategic Planning for Nurses, Organization Environment Relationships,* and *Just a Nurse.*

Marilyn J. Rantz, M.S.N., R.N., is Administrator of Lakeland Nursing Home of Walworth County, Elkhorn, Wisconsin, and a doctoral nursing student at the University of Wisconsin-Milwaukee.

Janet Wessel Krejci, M.S., R.N., is Adjunct Assistant Professor of Nursing at Marquette University in Milwaukee, and a doctoral candidate at the University of Wisconsin-Milwaukee.

Library of Congress Cataloging-in-Publication Data

Quality of health care for older people in America : a review of
  nursing studies / Norma M. Lang ... [et al.].
    p. cm.
  Includes bibliographical references.
  ISBN 1-55810-060-1 (pbk., perfectbound)
  1. Geriatric nusing. 2. Aged—Care—United States. I. Lang,
Norma M.
  [DNLM: 1. Aged.   2. Geriatric Nursing.   3. Quality of Health Care.
WY 152 Q2]
RC954.Q35 1990
362.1'9897'00973—dc20
DNLM/DLC
for Library of Congress   91-4547
                                                              CIP

Published by
American Nurses Association
2420 Pershing Road
Kansas City, Missouri 64108

GE-13   1M   12/90

Contents

Tables

Section 5

Preface

Almost three million registered nurses provide care to patients in virtually every type of health care setting in this country. Nursing therapies have a major impact on the effectiveness of health care and the costs of that care, especially in care systems outside of the hospital. A large portion of the nation's health care patients are elderly Medicare beneficiaries or recipients. Yet, nursing care of the elderly is relatively invisible when it comes to public policy, and related nursing research often is overlooked.

This publication is a response to that situation. It should reassure and energize all nurses through its clear demonstration of the substantial nursing contributions to the advancement of health sciences.

Nurses working with the elderly in clinical settings will find that this report summarizes various nurse-managed intervention programs that have significantly improved the health statuses of elderly persons. Many studies validate that the competencies of nursing staff and their effects on patient processes and outcomes are major indicators of quality of health care in hospitals, home care programs, and nursing homes. This report also summarizes many care problems nurses face daily and indicates care modalities which could benefit from further testing and validation in practice.

Politically active nurses interested in influencing public policy will find that this report documents the valuable contributions of nurses to the continued search for quality of care for the nation's elderly. The Robert Wood Johnson Foundation Teaching Nursing Home Program (Small and Walsh, 1988), for example, shows how nursing positively affects care processes and outcomes—resulting in reduced use of hospital care and shortened lengths of stay in nursing homes. With regard to home health services, research demonstrates that routine monitoring of older persons in their homes decreases the incidence of hospitalization and can increase independence. This kind of nursing care, however, is not a reimbursable service.

Additionally, graduate students and nurse researchers can use the bibliography and research summaries in this report as valuable starting points for their scholarly explorations.

The opportunity to produce this report presented itself when Rubenstein, Rubenstein, and Josephson submitted their review of recently published research on the *Quality of Health Care for Older People in America* to the Institute of Medicine in February 1989. Nursing research was totally absent from the summary of 226 studies that focused on the quality of medical care for the elderly. In fact, the authors commented that "nonphysician care is extremely important in determining outcomes of care for geriatric patients. *Yet, the quality of nursing care,* physical and occupational therapy care, and social work care are *virtually unstudied* [emphasis added]."

In response, a team of nursing faculty members and doctoral students at the University of Wisconsin-Milwaukee School of Nursing immediately began to review published gerontological nursing research—ultimately reviewing more than 4,000 published papers. Approximately 400 of these papers were referenced in another report on the *Quality of Health Care for Older People in America* by Lang and Kraegel, which was submitted to the Institute of Medicine in June 1989 as a companion report to the Rubenstein, Rubenstein, and Josephson paper. Clearly, the quality of health care of the elderly has received considerable research attention from nurses.

Readers are cautioned, however, to bear in mind that the selections in this publication are by no means exhaustive. For example, there are dozens of published studies on decubiti, confusion, and self-care. The citations herein were selected to describe research findings relevant to the quality of care of the elderly from a nursing perspective. Additionally, the methodology used to locate these studies (described in Section 1) was not all-encompassing—it was chosen to parallel the Rubenstein, Rubenstein, and Josephson approach. This methodology also allowed the nurse researchers working on this report to complete the original review within the tight deadlines imposed by the Institute of Medicine for consideration of papers.

This report was a group effort made on behalf of the nursing profession to examine the status of nursing research regarding the quality of health care for the elderly. Rantz and Krejci joined Lang and Kraegel in revising the original report for publication. Approximately 100 more recent nursing research studies focusing on care of the elderly that were published in 1989-90 have been added to the original bibliography. Due to numerous nursing requests for portions of the paper, the authors decided to publish this material through the American Nurses Association, and will direct any royalties earned to the American Nurses Foundation—to be earmarked for nursing research projects. With these steps, the authors hope to further research efforts of interest to nursing and to the American public. □

Acknowledgements

The individuals responsible for the development of this material collectively contributed their expertise and time because of their commitment to nursing and geriatric health care services. Dr. Norma Lang provided the spark one evening in a graduate quality assurance nursing class. She felt that the addition of nursing's research contributions could strengthen a research report on quality of health care for older people which had been commissioned by the Institutes of Medicine—four doctoral students met with her after class and resolved to organize a nursing reply. Two other doctoral students and Dr. Janet Kraegel later joined the group. This publication is the outcome of their efforts.

Janet Kraegel synthesized the clusters of studies and wrote the body of the paper with Norma Lang.

Marilyn Rantz organized the abstracting efforts, abstracted research articles, and coded and categorized the abstracts for the report. She later updated the report by abstracting additional research articles, revising the charts, and cross-referencing the bibliographies for publication.

Janet Wessel Krejci was Dr. Lang's research assistant at the time this project was undertaken. She abstracted articles from *Dissertation Abstracts,* developed the original charts, and assisted with editing the original report.

The authors would like to extend special appreciation to the following individuals for assistance in the development of this material:

Mary Zwygart-Stauffacher, M.S.N., R.N., C., is a gerontological nurse practitioner and a doctoral candidate at the University of Wisconsin-Milwaukee. She abstracted several journal articles, reviewed nursing textbooks, and prepared the material for Section 6.

Karen Marek, M.S.N., R.N., is a doctoral candidate at the University of Wisconsin-Milwaukee and a graduate assistant to Dr. Lang. She abstracted several journals and facilitated the group's efforts.

Bonnie Westra, M.S.N., R.N., is a doctoral candidate at the University of Wisconsin-Milwaukee and a consultant in home care in Rochester, Minnesota. She abstracted several journals, facilitated the efforts of other group members, and critiqued the research categorizations.

Amy Coenon, M.S.N., R.N., is a doctoral nursing student at the University of Wisconsin-Milwaukee and the Quality Assurance Coordinator at Milwaukee County Mental Health Complex. She abstracted several articles and facilitated the group's efforts.

Finally, special thanks to clinical specialists Jane Wall and Marie Maguire of Lakeland Nursing Home for their abstracting efforts, and to Lynda Badertscher for her typing and project follow-up. □

1

Introduction

Purpose

This report is a critical review of published literature
on the quality of health care for the elderly population in the
United States, from the perspective of clinical geriatric/
gerontological nursing. It is a companion report to the
February 1, 1989 Rubenstein, Rubenstein, and Josephson
paper prepared for the Institute of Medicine. Therefore, the
same general format of the Rubenstein, Rubenstein, and
Josephson review has been retained.

The Rubenstein, Rubenstein, and Josephson paper's
purpose was to present "a critical review of the published
literature on the quality of *medical* care for the elderly population in the United States from the perspective of clinical
geriatric medicine [emphasis added]." The nursing
perspective of this report, however, requires a broader
understanding of the terms *health* and *quality* than does
the Rubenstein, Rubenstein, and Josephson paper, even
though both reports are subsumed under the title "Quality
of Health Care for Older People in America."

The Rubenstein, Rubenstein, and Josephson paper suggests that data sources for quality assessment for the elderly
should include nonphysician members of the multidisciplinary team and may require emphasis on diseases and conditions that must use rehabilitation, social work, and home
care services. As a direct response to that suggestion, the
focus of this paper includes nurse value-based definitions of
health and *quality* that include disease prevention, health

maintenance, rehabilitation, costs, environmental safety, self-care, and quality of life issues. However, literature reviews of social work, physical therapy, occupational therapy, and other health disciplines are still missing.

The essential difference between the Rubenstein, Rubenstein, and Josephson paper and this one is best exemplified by Shanas (1974), who notes that there are two major approaches to health status assessments among the elderly—the medical model, which stresses the importance of physical examination, and the functional model, which relies on functional status. Different interpretations of health resulting from the application of these two models reflect that the medical model is based on absolute levels of health (i.e., morbidity and mortality), rather than on levels of health relative to one's age and sex.

In the Rubenstein, Rubenstein, and Josephson paper, functionality or health status indicators of the elderly are not addressed directly, with the exception of Table 4.1, which lists nine medical studies on functional status related to processes of confusion, falling, eating, and incontinence in acute care settings. However, these functional states are the basis for nursing care and outcome requirements and the corresponding costs for that care.

The term "functional states," as understood by nursing, includes the physical, psychological, and social parameters that enable people to maintain or improve their state of health and experience quality of life.

The Rubenstein, Rubenstein, and Josephson paper acknowledges that functional status-related processes do have an effect on the costs of care and overall client perception of independence, health, and quality of life; their paper also expresses regret over the paucity of literature in this area. These are the very areas that are present in the nursing literature. Quality of life, self-care abilities, independence, confusion, skin integrity, mobility, eating, peaceful death, emotional well-being, autonomy, continence, and caregiver support are some of the care phenomena of concern to nurses. Unquestionably, these aspects of patient care influence the costs of health care, but are not made as explicit as the cost of a surgical procedure or laboratory test. In addition, these aspects influence the client's perception of quality of health care.

The incidence of chronic disease increases with aging. Chronic disease often results in loss of function and an increased dependency—an expensive proposition for the individual and his/her family, as well as for society. This study of nursing literature emphasizes research that describes nursing interventions for older populations to prevent iatrogenesis, and to maintain or restore function within a framework encompassing the physical, psychological, social, and economic needs of the elderly.

Health care for the elderly covers a wide range of services that affect the elderly's chronic conditions, disabilities, and dependent states. The aims of such services are:

- maintenance or improvement of health status,
- increase in self-care abilities,
- modification of the environment to eliminate physical and psychological barriers to desired autonomy,
- maintenance of quality of life, and
- achievement of a peaceful death.

The majority of the nursing literature in this study focuses on quality measures within this broad scope of health services. Outcomes measure a combination of patient, nursing, medical, rehabilitation, and social parameters and values.

In keeping with the format of the Rubenstein, Rubenstein, and Josephson paper, nursing literature on underuse and overuse of health services by the elderly is described under those section headings. Nursing research, however, is not customarily designed to identify care deficiencies in large populations; rather, the vast majority of nursing research is directed toward developing screening and assessment tools and testing nursing therapy techniques and outcomes for the elderly.

In contrast to the discussion in the Rubenstein, Rubenstein, and Josephson paper of medical screening, utilization of high technology, and physician management of disease conditions, the foci of this paper are nursing assessments, nursing interventions, and patient outcomes resulting from nursing practice.

Method

The given time frame of six weeks in which to generate this report necessitated an expedient and nonexhaustive study of the published literature. Furthermore, research related to the quality of nursing care of the elderly appears under many search descriptors in the health literature. Therefore, a broad approach was used to locate relevant publications. Journals of general nursing, quality assurance, nursing research, and nursing gerontology published in the last 10 years were selected and reviewed by five doctoral students. Through careful study of the journals' tables of contents, the students identified titles relating to clinical gerontological nursing research.

In addition, bibliographic lists were solicited from gerontological nursing faculty. *Dissertation Abstracts* (1983-1989) and chapters in the *Annual Review of Nursing Research* (1983-1989) also were reviewed. Finally, several nurse researchers throughout the United States were contacted to request their most relevant references on quality of care for the elderly. Table 1.1 contains a summary of journals, the number of articles searched, and the number of those included in this report. All research articles that contained data pertaining to issues of quality of care for the elderly from the perspective of clinical gerontological nursing were included in this review. Most articles focused on populations over age 65. Non-nursing journals reviewed in the Rubenstein, Rubenstein, and Josephson paper were not reviewed again.

The nursing doctoral students selected the initial list of journal articles; conducted a secondary review of the abstracted articles; and coded them by relevance, setting, and category. *Relevance* meant that the study provided data useful to the quality of care for the elderly. *Settings* were identified as hospitals, nursing homes, clients' homes, outpatient facilities, subacute hospital wards (i.e., rehabilitation), community/elderly housing, long-term care facilities, or outpatient day care programs. *Categories* included underuse, overuse, technical quality of care, and intervention programs.

The Rubenstein, Rubenstein, and Josephson paper rated the strength of the literature selections according to four categories used by the Canadian Task Force on the Periodic Health Examination (1979) to grade the effectiveness of a diagnostic test. The criteria indicate a bias toward tightly-controlled multisite experimental studies, and fail to acknowledge the equally vital qualitative, descriptive, quasi-experimental, and meta-analytical research methodologies used to empirically describe the health statuses, behaviors, and health outcomes of people. In this nursing research report, theoretical and opinion articles were deleted. Research articles that were included, if they were data-based, had a clearly-described sampling procedure and used methodology appropriate to the research question.

Each section in this part of the report is presented in two

parts. In the first part, the section topic is described in narrative form. Each narrative section is followed by a table that contains a selection of studies. Specific studies are not cited in the narrative; groups of studies are discussed in general. This method is congruent with the Rubenstein, Rubenstein, and Josephson paper. Each table contains a) selected studies, with a brief description of the study population, type of design, and findings; and b) a list of other references for the topic.

This nursing report also includes a bibliography presented in two formats—the first is presented alphabetically; the second is presented by 35 quality of care research areas. An effort was made to cross-index studies in the bibliography and the 35 tables which may have relevance to more than one research area. [Table 1.2 contains a summary of the quality of care research areas and number of selected studies.] □

Table 1.1
SUMMARY OF JOURNALS REVIEWED AND TECHNIQUES USED TO IDENTIFY QUALITY OF CARE PAPERS

Identification Technique	Approximate Number of Papers Published (1980-1990)	Approximate Number of Papers Selected
A. Journals reviewed for papers relevant to quality of care for elderly people		
• Research in Nursing & Health	321	36
• Image	211	7
• Western Journal of Nursing Research	317	5
• Nursing Research	511	55
• Quality Review Bulletin	555	34
• Issues in Mental Health Nursing	133	3
• Archives of Psychiatric Nursing	165	10
• Journal of Gerontological Nursing	501	128
• Geriatric Nursing	417	44
• American Journal of Nursing	1189	8
• Advances in Nursing Science	102	12
• Nursing and Health Care	336	3
B. Additional papers and selected research-based book chapters identified by hand search, personal contact, and bibliography review		77
C. Dissertation abstracts		54
TOTALS	4758	476

Note: Due to availability of journals, not all issues were obtained.

Table 1.2
SUMMARY OF QUALITY OF CARE RESEARCH AREAS AND NUMBERS OF SELECTED STUDIES

Topic of Quality of Care Research	Number of Studies Selected
• Underuse of Services by Older People	N = 15
• Overuse of Services by Older People	N = 32
• Technical Quality of Care: Patient/Client-Focused Issues	
Quality of Life, Life Satisfaction, and Health Promotion	N = 51
Mental Health of Older People	N = 33
Relaxation and Multimethod Nursing Therapies	N = 8
Self-Care and Activities of Daily Living	N = 20
Physiological Health of Older People	
Food and Fluid Intake, Oral Hygiene	N = 15
Nocturnal Behavior	N = 4
Incontinence	N = 22
Pressure Sores	N = 16
Thermoregulation and Cardiovascular Parameters	N = 17
Exercise	N = 10
Foot Care	N = 5
Cognitive Function	
Health Teaching	N = 8
Confusion	N = 28
Psychosocial Health Dysfunction	
Bereavement	N = 13
Relocation	N = 10
Issues Surrounding Quality of Death: End-of-Life Directives	N = 7
• Technical Quality of Care: Family-Focused Issues	
Family Caregiver Issues	N = 22
Nursing Home Placement Decision Criteria	N = 15
• Technical Quality of Care: Nursing Staff Issues	N = 34
• Intervention Programs to Improve the Quality of Geriatric Care	
Quality Assurance Programs	N = 10
Examples of Quality Assurance Tools	N = 9
Programs Which Improve the Effectiveness of Health Care	N = 19
Fall Prevention Programs:	
Examples of Fall Prevention Programs	N = 7
Risk Factors of Elderly Who Fall	N = 8
Intervention Programs to Improve the Mental Status	
of the Cognitively Impaired Elderly	N = 38
	T = 476

2

Underuse of services by older people

The Rubenstein, Rubenstein, and Josephson paper defines *underuse* in terms of underdiagnosis and under-treatment. *Nursing services,* per se, remain undefined throughout the paper. Nursing services include actual physical and mental care, health teaching, health promotion, disease prevention, health screening, health care management, the fostering of self-care, family support, and administration of medical treatments. Nurses administer and monitor medical regimens, conduct physical assessments, plan and evaluate care, and coordinate multiple health care resources for elderly patients. Nurses provide the majority of care within hospitals, nursing homes, home care programs, ambulatory care settings, day care programs, and public health services. Increasingly, nurses are providing care for the elderly in ambulatory clinics and high-rise residential living centers.

Access to care is a term frequently contained in definitions of quality. In the case of home care nursing services, *lack of access to nursing care by the elderly* may be a better descriptor than *underuse* (see Tables 2.1 to 2.3). Access to care is determined by *medical necessity* and medical referrals for home care. Criteria used to determine medical necessity do not adequately cover nursing necessity. Categorizing nursing care under medical diagnosis and necessity, especially in long-term care situations, and using only technical treatment terms (i.e., intravenous therapy, indwelling catheter, and respiratory dependency) leaves large care deficits and inadequate data bases to remedy the deficits.

Several studies (see Table 2.1) examined the responses of elderly patients to home care nursing. These studies indicated that elderly home care patients lacked knowledge about availability of services and the referral process. The amount and intensity of services have a significant influence on improving the physical functioning of elderly patients at safe, acceptable levels. However, many are forced to stop the services prematurely because Medicare benefits have run out.

Mortality rates and hospitalization rates are found to increase when the home health services of nursing, medical treatment, and homemaking are no longer available to patients. One descriptive study documented that following the implementation of diagnosis-related group (DRG) classifications, patients receiving home care were more severely ill, yet the number of home health care visits did not rise to compensate for increased severity.

The living arrangements, functional statuses, and gender of the elderly significantly influence consumption levels of Medicare-reimbursed home health services. Older females receive fewer home visits by professionals and more visits by nonprofessionals than do older males, yet females have higher levels of functional impairment and fewer available caretakers (see Table 2.2).

In terms of underdiagnosis and undertreatment, women in one comparison study received less timely diagnoses and less vigorous treatments for lung cancer than did men. In another study of gynecological screening conducted by nurses, 52% of the elderly women had one or more abnormalities which required physician follow-up, even though 83% of these women had been seen by a physician within the previous year. Elderly patients of both sexes have less analgesic medicine prescribed and administered postoperatively than do younger patients. Further study is needed to determine levels of acceptable pain relief.

Underdiagnosis of cognitive impairment in the elderly is a situation of major concern (see Table 2.3). Successful rehabilitation of persons with chronic diseases is predicated on the patients' abilities to receive information and to learn and maintain a medical and self-care regimen.

In a study of 182 elderly admitted to an acute care hospital, 47 had significant cognitive deficits which were undetected during the routine admission assessment procedure. These findings have serious implications for the safety of elderly patients, both within the hospital and following discharge. According to three studies, 25%-43% of those released from hospitals following a serious illness had problems following their medically-prescribed regimens, and approximately 66% had difficulty with activities of daily living. Medicare benefits for home care are available only if the discharged patient is homebound and requires medically-determined treatment for a changing medical condition. Better descriptors are needed for skilled nursing care, including self-care teaching and monitoring and nursing care of chronic conditions. These descriptors, however, have limited Medicare coverage.

One study documented that deterioration of the condition of hospitalized patients was more directly related to age and abnormal mental status than to the intensity of medical treatment. This deterioration was thought to be related directly to the need for nursing care. Studies are needed in order to measure deterioration that can be prevented by medical and nursing therapies, and deterioration that requires high-quality supportive care at an acceptable cost.

These 15 nursing studies on underuse are similar to those described in the Rubenstein, Rubenstein, and Josephson paper in that they are descriptive and limited to the establishment of correlations, not causality. As strongly indicated in the Rubenstein, Rubenstein, and Josephson paper, the elderly fail to receive the quantity and quality of health care they need for restoration of function, maintenance of safety, and prevention of rehospitalization.   □

Table 2.1
UNDERUSE: HOME HEALTH (Selected References)

Reference	Study Population	Design	Findings
Gorenberg (1986)	N = 45 frail elderly patients, ages 74+, discharged from home service	Descriptive study to examine consequences of discharge from home care of frail elderly	Amount & intensity of service has significant influence on improved physical functioning; need for services varies little over time; financial ability to maintain services drops postdischarge
Card (1987)	N = 54 patients referred for home care	Descriptive study of patient satisfaction with home health nursing service; patient knowledge	Underutilization, overall few minorities; little collaboration between health care providers
Preston & Grimes (1987)	N = 900 elderly in community ages 65-94	Descriptive study to identify needs of community	Only 4% of sample used agency help; more social support needed
Moyer (1987)	N = 58 elderly discharged from Medicare home health "stable"	Descriptive study to examine quality of recidivism & death related to spouse caregiving	Significant relationship between time spouse gave care & rehospitalization; 10% mortality, 20% rehospitalization for all elderly
Wolock, Schlesinger, Dinerman, & Seaton (1987)	N = 69 elderly hospitalized for serious illnesses, ages 60 and over	Descriptive study to identify needs related to activities of daily living (ADL) regime	Family major caregiver; ⅔ had difficulty with ADL; 53% deteriorated; 25-43% had trouble following regime; many stopped services as benefits ended (medicine, 25%; nursing, 41%)

Other references in this area: (Bredow, 1989; Feldman, Weiss, & Small, 1989; VanOrt & Woodtli, 1989)

Table 2.2
UNDERUSE: ELDERLY WOMEN (Selected References)

Reference	Study Population	Design	Findings
Pasquale (1987)	N = 100 random, mean age 76 years, community home health	Descriptive study to identify utilization related to functional impairment and gender	Older women received fewest nursing visits and highest nonprofessional visits, yet had the greatest functional impairment
Packard (1988)	N = 89	Descriptive study of variables associated with health care utilization	Males had significantly higher number of treatments than women; MD specialty and early treatment effort were best predictors of later hospital use
Denny, Koren, & Wisby (1989)	N = 62, ages 60-85	Descriptive study of elderly women to identify gynecological health issues	Over half of women were found to have one or more gynecologic abnormalities, despite that all saw MD within previous year

Table 2.3
UNDERUSE: DIAGNOSIS (Selected References)

Reference	Study Population	Design	Findings
Faherty & Grier (1984)	N = 772, stratified by sex into 10-year groupings, random sample of 142	Experimental design, 7 groups to test effect of age on postoperative medication	Older patients had less analgesic medication prescribed and administered postoperatively
Palmateer & McCartney (1985)	N = 182 elderly hospitalized during 6-week period	Quasi-experimental design to test systematic assessments related to confusion	Those assessed with Systematic Cognitive Tool had better percentage of being recognized and treated

Other references in this area: (Reed & Birge, 1988; Scura & Wipple, 1990)

SECTION

3

Overuse of services by older people

Definitions of quality of health care, at the very minimum, contain the dimensions of timely and appropriate care at the least cost. Once hospitalized, older patients are medically diagnosed and treated, and rarely remain in the hospital unless nursing care is required. Nurses, therefore, have a key responsibility for assuring that appropriate care takes place in a timely manner with no iatrogenic occurrences. From a nursing perspective, overuse of institutional resources (hospitals and nursing homes) by the elderly is frequently the result of:

- insufficient planning, nursing surveillance and therapy, and coordination of care;
- inappropriate hospitalization; and
- insufficient teaching of self-care competencies to the elderly and their caregivers.

Nurses are responsible for conducting initial assessments of patients' responses to medical and other health care therapies, and elderly persons' self-care competencies, their coping strategies, and the context in which they function. Nurses develop care and discharge plans, schedule other health provider services, deliver nursing services, procure services, monitor care, evaluate the adequacy of services, teach the elderly and their caregivers, and maintain a safe environment for patients.

The 32 nursing studies on overuse of services primarily contained questions about the extent to which overuse of hospitals and nursing homes could be curtailed (see Tables 3.1 to 3.4). It was found, for instance, that when nurses conducted hospital discharge planning at the time of admission for patients who were being treated for one of five chronic disease conditions, the length of stay decreased .8 days (2 days for stroke patients). For every day that discharge planning was postponed, the length of stay increased .8 days. Patients being discharged to nursing homes stayed in the hospital 10-12 days longer than did patients discharged to their homes (see Table 3.1).

A separate descriptive study found that the savings for 80 hospitalized persons over age 75 was $34,707—due to reduced lengths of stay when a gerontological clinical nurse specialist was able to conduct an initial assessment and assisted with coordination of services. Similarly, when nurses conducted intensive health promotion activities with 43 elderly persons with circulation disturbances in their lower extremities, lengths of stay were reduced by 8.24 days and costs were reduced by $112,387, compared to a control group that did not take part in the program.

In a study of 1,255 medical-surgical patients up to 97 years of age, the patients' dependence on nursing care explained 58.98% of the variance in length of stay, compared to 11.12% of the variance explained by medical diagnosis. Similarly, a study of severity of illness in patients with myocardial infarction found that severity of illness is a better predictor of nursing costs than the ICD-9-CM system (International Classification of Diseases, 9th edition, Clinical Modification) and DRG classifications. These findings raise validity questions about the use of medical DRG (diagnosis-related groups) diagnoses to regulate the lengths of stay for hospitalized patients, especially the elderly.

In a study of long-term care facilities, findings indicated that a nursing diagnosis of patients' dependence on nursing care was a better indicator of lengths of stay than the medical problem list. Nursing problems are amenable to nursing interventions, whereas medical diagnoses of the elderly often mean irreversible conditions. For instance, when third-party payers reimbursed 34 hospitals and four rural health centers for the services of a nurse diabetic educator, the hospitals experienced a 32.2% reduction in their admissions of diabetic patients (see Table 3.2).

One study demonstrated that routine weekly visits by a

community health nurse decreased the incidence of hospitalization for older persons. Another study showed that a nurse practitioner assigned to the elderly population living in a high rise could effectively assess, monitor, and maintain their health statuses and independence with the help of a home health aide for the 32% requiring assistance with activities of daily living. A third study verified that elderly patients who used nurse-managed clinics for their health problems experienced a hospitalization rate lower than the national average.

In a study of reactions of the elderly toward nurses performing primary care functions, the majority either preferred the nurse or had no preference for being seen by a physician. As a group, results of these studies indicate that nurses can reduce the overuse of expensive hospitalization and improve patients' health outcomes when the nurses' care planning and health promotion skills are fully utilized.

Nursing studies substantiated the Rubenstein, Rubenstein, and Josephson paper's conclusion that the elderly receive an excess amount of drugs (see Table 3.3). Research indicates that patients followed by nurse practitioners use fewer drugs than patients followed by physicians. In a controlled study of the routine use of neuroleptic medication in a nursing home, those receiving the medication displayed more significant behavioral excesses and had a higher rate of physical and motor symptoms than those matched for mental status who were placed in the no-drug group.

A second nursing home successfully instituted a one-day-a-week drug "holiday," which resulted in a 9% reduction in drug consumption without untoward results. Similarly, in a study in which digoxin was withdrawn from nine patients ages 82 to 95, six did not require further use of the drug. Further multidisciplinary research is needed for the most effective medication regimes for elderly nursing home residents. Record audits of 102 nursing home patients in three facilities revealed that 71% regularly received sleeping medications. This suggests that physicians and nurses are unaware of the normal changes in sleep patterns which accompany the aging process. Most prescribed sleeping medications are administered at the discretion of the nursing staff.

An issue not addressed by the Rubenstein, Rubenstein, and Josephson study is the underuse of hospitals and the overuse of nursing home facilities for the care of acutely ill elderly patients. This situation is a result of the implementation of prospective payment systems (PPS). Five nursing studies documented an increase in the amount and complexity of care in nursing homes following PPS implementation (see Table 3.4).

Nurse administrators in 25 nursing homes reported that the increased acuity of patients following DRG policy implementation required changes in nurses' work loads, staffing patterns, and staff development programs. Record audits in a study of 120 nursing home Medicare patients demonstrated a significant increase in total nursing care requirements following PPS implementation. A comparison of pre-DRG and post-DRG admissions conducted in another skilled nursing facility evidenced that the post-DRG group required twice the number of nursing actions in the first three days as compared to the pre-DRG group. If reimbursement mechanisms do not keep pace with the requirements for additional intense and sophisticated therapies and increased patient monitoring in nursing homes and home care situations, the overall quality of care deteriorates for all residents and patients.   □

Table 3.1
OVERUSE: LENGTH OF STAY (Selected References)

Reference	Study Population	Design	Findings
Leslie (1981)	N = 210 elderly in long-term care	Comparative analysis of medical and nursing diagnosis & the relation of each to subsequent direction for care	Nursing diagnosis found to be more comprehensive and indicative of care than medical diagnosis; medical diagnoses referred to irreversible conditions, where nursing diagnoses were amenable to intervention
Ventura, Young, Feldman, Pastore, Pidula, & Yates (1985)	N = 86 random assignment, arterial insufficiency	Experimental design to examine cost-effectiveness of nursing intervention to promote patient involvement	Treatment group had significantly shorter lengths of stay, significantly lower hospital costs, and increased health outcomes
Marchette & Holloman (1986)	N = 100 stratified random sample for 5 chronic conditions	Retrospective experimental design using multiple regression to examine impact related to RN discharge planning	When RN did discharge planning, decrease of .8 day of stay; 2-day decrease for cardiovascular patient; for each day discharge planning delayed, increase of .8 day of hospital stay
Neidlinger, Scoggins, & Kennedy (1987)	N = 80 random	Double-blind experimental study utilizing control group and Comprehensive Discharge Planning Protocol with gerontological clinical nurse specialist prepared at the master's degree level	Significantly lower costs for group receiving comprehensive discharge planning
Nosek (1987)	N = 1255 elderly medical/surgical patients at university hospital	Secondary analysis to examine influence on lengths of stay	Nursing diagnosis explained 59.8% of variance; medical diagnosis explained 11.12% of variance

Other references in this area: (Edwardson, 1988; Grau & Kobner, 1986; Hobler & Howlett, 1985; Hogan & Smith, 1987; Lamont, Sampson, Matthias, & Kane, 1983; Micheletti & Shlala, 1986)

Table 3.2
OVERUSE: HOSPITALIZATION AND COSTS (Selected References)

Reference	Study Population	Design	Findings
Thorbury & Martin (1983)	N = 20 elderly home health clients	Quasi-experimental design to examine impact of nursing visits	Group that did not see RN on weekly basis had higher incidence of hospitalization and higher costs
Schwartz, Zaremba, & Ra (1985)	N = 24 hospitals, 4 rural health centers, & 1 home health	Pre-test & posttest design; 1:1 and group teaching with diabetic clinical nurse educator	There was a 32.2% decrease in the number of hospitalizations, as well as a decrease in costs
Igou, Hawkins, Johnson, & Utely (1989)	N = 75 clients, majority over age 70; 679 nurse practitioner visits	Posttest design assessing impact on hospitalization rate and lengths of stay in patients seen by a nurse practitioner	Hospitalization rate and lengths of stay lower than national average; 78 referrals made—35 to MDs
Kline (1989)	N = 109; cross-section of 51 females, 58 males; mean age 65, with chronic obstructive pulmonary disease	Cross-sectional survey to examine correlates of disease severity and basic need satisfaction, perceived stress, gender, & other variables, & interaction effects	Disease severity, need satisfaction, & gender all had significant effect on illness symptoms; direction for nursing intervention to decrease symptoms & lengths of stay

Other references in this area: (Collard, 1989; Cleveland, 1988; Brands, 1983; Collard, Bachman, & Beatrice, 1985; Ventura, Young, Feldman, Pastore, Pidula, & Yates, 1984)

Table 3.3
OVERUSE: RESTRAINT AND MEDICATION USAGE (Selected References)

Reference	Study Population	Design	Findings
Keenan, Redshaw, Munson, & Mundt (1983)	Long-term care patients	Descriptive pilot study of drug holiday 1 day per week	No change in cardiac status, with 9% decrease in drug consumption; savings of $4600
Chisolm, Lundin, & Wood (1983)	N = 9 elderly on digoxin	Quasi-experimental design related to withdrawal of digoxin	⅔ (6) did not need digoxin on 2-month or 10-month follow-up
Clapin-French (1986)	N = 102 elderly in long-term care	Descriptive study of sleep patterns and medication use	71% of patients on sleep medication; medication use not necessarily related to identified need
Butler, Burgio, & Engel (1987)	N = 60 random elderly patients with dementia	Experimental 2-group post-test: those receiving routine neuroleptics with matched group receiving no neuroleptic medication	Patients receiving neuroleptic medications had significantly more behavioral, gastrointestinal, & central nervous system problems
Strumpf & Evans (1988)	N = 20 medical patients, mean age 73.3, frail elderly	Descriptive study of restraint use; interview patients & nurses	Patients expressed anger, discomfort, fear, & resistance; nurses expressed conflict of protective needs of patient and own professional values of nonrestrictive environment
Brown & Everett (1990)	N = 41 elderly in long-term care hospital ward	Experimental, with control group	39% fewer doses of bowel medications; 43% cost savings with fiber supplement vs. bowel medications

Table 3.4
OVERUSE: DRG-RELATED STUDIES (Selected References)

Reference	Study Population	Design	Findings
Harron & Schaeffer (1986)	N = 100 skilled nursing care patients coming from hospitals prior to and following implementation of diagnosis-related groups (DRG)	Descriptive design comparison of outcomes prior to and following implementation of prospective payment systems (PPS)	Patients admitted to long-term facility post-DRG needed significantly more nursing and complex care; pre-DRG, 195 interventions in first 3 days; post-DRG, 405 nursing interventions in first 3 days
Stull & Vernon (1986)	N = 25 administrative nurses from skilled long-term care facilities	Descriptive design interviews to ascertain changes in work load, staff development needs, and organizational policies post-DRG	Significant increase in all variables post-DRG in skilled long-term care
Gamroth (1988)	N = 120 medical records from 2 long-term care facilities; randomly selected in 3 categories: cardiovascular, hip fracture, & miscellaneous	Descriptive design comparison of pre-PPS and post-PPS related to specific variables	Lengths of stay in hospital decreased significantly; no change in lengths of stay in nursing homes, but significant increase in nursing requirements, nursing interventions, and number of medications used under PPS
Fitzgerald, Moore, & Dittus (1988) [physician study]	N = 560 elderly patients with hip fracture, over age 65	Descriptive (retrospective) examining of outcomes of PPS	Since PPS hospitals have reduced amount of care given, there are increasing lengths of stay in nursing homes, as well as number of patients remaining in nursing homes

Other references in this area: (McGovern & Newbern, 1988; Weinberg, Engingro, Miller, Weinberg, & Parker, 1989)

4

Technical quality of care for older people

Introduction

There has been formal interest in the assessment and
assurance of the quality of nursing care since 1858, when
Florence Nightingale used a set of standards to assess the
care provided during the Crimean War. Objective and sys-
tematic evaluation of nursing care has continued to be a
priority within the nursing profession. For a more extensive
review of the literature, the reader is referred to Lang's
*Nurse Planning Series Volume 12, Quality Assurance in Nurs-
ing: A Selected Bibliography* (Lang, 1980), which contains
367 abstracts classified according to foci of the studies.

One hundred sixty-four research reports assessing the
quality of nursing care from 1974 to 1982 can be found in
volume 2, chapter 6 of *Annual Review of Nursing Research*
(1984). The authors (Lang and Clinton, 1984) used a struc-
ture-process-outcome framework to review published
empirical studies of assessment of the quality of nursing
care. [Most nursing authors use the structure-process-out-
come framework proposed by Donabedian (1980).]

The intent of this section is to make inferences from the
geriatric/gerontological nursing literature about processes
and outcomes that should be used in quality assurance
activities for older people, and to identify the most common
nursing deficiencies in health care of the elderly. The
authors agree with the Rubenstein, Rubenstein, and

Josephson paper's finding that more published data-based, geriatric quality of care studies are needed, and also agree that the interest demonstrated by researchers in particular processes and outcomes reflects their clinical importance and measurement feasibility. The authors believe that a very large but unknown number of research and evaluation projects to assess the quality of care were never published.

The nursing processes and patient outcomes described herein have been measured using record audits or commonly accepted research instruments applied to elderly populations in community acute care hospitals and long-term care settings. This section is organized around issues focused on the patient, the family, and nursing staffing. Each of these issues influences quality of health care for the elderly. A general discussion of each issue is followed by a table of selected specific studies.

Patient/Client-Focused Issues

The focus in this critical review of published nursing literature on the quality of care of the elderly is *health,* especially those aspects of health influenced by nursing care. This integrated perspective extends beyond medicine's focus on the absence or presence of disease, or the ability to carry out one's role in life. It encompasses assistance of the elderly in adjusting to their health states within the context of their families, environments, and life-styles. Nursing care of the elderly is predicated on the beliefs that the patient is capable of making gains necessary to meet mutually-established health goals; that the endeavor is a worthwhile process; and that older persons, in most cases, can make their own choices if they receive appropriate information.

Quality of Life, Life Satisfaction, and Health Promotion

The 51 selected nursing studies on health values, health promotion activities, and health perceptions of the elderly validate that the majority of elderly have positive health values and participate in health promotion activities to a greater extent than do their younger counterparts (see Table 4.1). One study supports the statement that participation in health promotion activities is the best predictor for quality of life.

The Rubenstein, Rubenstein, and Josephson paper does not directly address the definition of *quality of health care,* which influenced their choice of literature to review. However, their choices reflect a focus on technically correct medical care which neither overutilizes nor underutilizes medical care resources.

Nursing definitions of *quality* center on whether expected patient outcomes (in terms of self-care and functional health status) are achieved in a cost-effective manner, and whether or not the client is satisfied with the care received. Ongoing arguments that patients lack the knowledge to evaluate technical aspects of care are supported. However, patients play an important role in defining what constitutes quality of care, since they determine what values should be associated with different outcomes (i.e., the end products of care).

Clinical geriatric/gerontological nursing research attempts to validate clients' beliefs, values, and satisfiers in order to provide health structures and processes that will produce valued outcomes for the elderly, especially those receiving long-term care. The literature reviewed in this section contains research on factors that affect perceptions of the elderly about health status, life satisfaction, and quality of life.

The research indicates that when the elderly have a positive outlook, they perceive themselves as having good health—despite chronic illness and social/physical limitations. Eleven nursing studies focused on quality of life and morale outcomes for older adults. Quality of life was significantly related to perceived health status, level of social activity, and ability to control one's life-style. The satisfaction of hemodialysis patients with their care correlated positively with their perceived quality of life.

There was a relationship between high morale and nursing home residents who perceived their admissions as voluntary, had social interaction, and had choices within the institution. Thirteen studies investigated life satisfaction of the elderly. Poor health status and loneliness had the strongest negative effects on this health status indicator. Three studies indicated that life satisfaction and morale are not significantly different for minority elderly and white elderly populations. Never-married older women were healthier, less lonely, and more positive than widows.

Four studies confirmed that life satisfaction correlated positively with a positive health perception and participation in health-promoting behaviors. In one study, path analysis was used to determine factors affecting the life satisfaction of nursing home residents. Health status, satisfaction with finances, and relationship with family were major variables affecting an elderly person's attitudes toward nursing homes.

Mental Health of Older People

According to the Federal Council on Aging, there are no hard data on the prevalence of mental health problems in the elderly. General estimates taken from a variety of sources indicate that 15-25% of the elderly living in communities have significant symptoms of mental illness, and 10% may experience clinically diagnosed depression. Among elderly nursing home residents, 16% have a primary diagnosis of senility.

About 40% of mental health disorders among the elderly are incorrectly diagnosed and treated. In addition to unnecessary psychological suffering, inadequate treatment leads to deterioration or complication of physical disorders, thereby increasing health care costs.

A meta-analysis of 41 experimental mental health studies concluded that therapy enhanced the mental health of clients. Therapy was defined as any nondrug treatment which nurses or other nonphysician health providers could be expected to control and use in their practice to relieve emotional distress and unacceptable behavior, enhance positive emotions, or increase cognitive skills.

Thirty-three clinical geriatric nursing studies examined mental health indices such as coping behaviors, social isolation, depression, and loneliness (see Table 4.2). The studies bear little relationship to each other, but indicate the nursing profession's recognition that mental health quality assessments of the elderly should extend beyond measurement of physical disease states, since good mental health improves physical health and vice versa. For instance, physical health status correlated negatively with degree of loneliness. In nursing homes, those residents who failed to thrive (i.e., inadequate intake) tended to be the most depressed, physically disabled, and cognitively disabled. Interestingly enough, in a matched comparison of healthy versus terminally ill adults, there was no difference in senses of well-being between the two groups.

Relaxation and Multimethod Nursing Therapies

Nurse researchers tested the outcomes of their practices in this review of the literature (see Table 4.3). One study documented physiological indicators of relaxation in nursing home patients following back rubs. Cachexia in at-risk cancer patients has been reversed by a combination of relaxation training, counseling, and nutritional supplementation. Visual imagery with music therapy significantly increased pain control and reduced chemotherapy-induced nausea and vomiting. Four hundred chemotherapy treatments administered to 71 home care patients by nurses resulted in a remarkable absence of nausea and vomiting and no infiltrations at the intravenous site.

Self-Care and Activities of Daily Living

Medical diagnoses poorly define the level and amount of health care services elderly patients require, either within institutions or in community health care settings. The decrease in loss of function and concomitant dependency associated with chronic diseases and the aging process require interdependent services which support and promote self-care. There has been considerable nursing research conducted on the self-care potential of elderly clients (see Table 4.4). In general, data suggest that improvement in self-care capacity not only results in psychological well-being of the elderly, but also extends survival.

One exploratory study resulted in an assessment profile that predicted those elderly clients with a high ability to assume self-care. An ethnographic study of nine discharged patients indicated that home health care may support dependency behavior as clients become well and capable of self-care—a finding that warrants further research. In a study of 563 patients discharged from nursing homes, only 28% were discharged to their homes. The best predictor of both immediate and two-year survival was their ability to assume activities of daily living. In a study of arthritic women, it was found that the combination of pain and difficulty in performing tasks eroded well-being. Similarly, a causal modeling research study indicated that control over activities of daily living was significantly related to well-being. In a related experimental study, there was a positive relationship between nursing home patients who dressed in their own clothes and levels of self-esteem and abilities to function.

Two studies used Framingham data to substantiate consequential impairment of stroke patients. Depression among stroke patients was four times more prevalent than it was in the Framingham control group, and a significant percentage of stroke survivors manifested continued social dysfunction despite complete physical restoration. The main predictor of institutionalization following strokes was dependence in activities of daily living. Another study of stroke patients indicated that recovery is more highly predicated on patients' cognitive and emotional coping skills than on physical predictors. This was corroborated by a separate exploratory study in which 29 stroke patients gained 72% in functioning at home and attributed 38% of their restoration to their families. Secondarily, physical environment barriers may impede home recovery.

Self-administration of medications is a major self-care concern of nurses. Four studies documented that noninstitutionalized elderly used over-the-counter drugs on a regular basis, and as many as 10% used medications prescribed from friends or family members. As many as 25% of the elderly exceeded recommended dosages for both over-the-counter and prescription drugs. Uncontrolled hypertensives had more complex medication regimens and lower compliance with self-medication than did controlled hypertensives. In general, the more prescriptions the elderly received, the greater their noncompliance with medication regimens.

Physiological Health of Older People

Physiological and cellular changes in the biological systems of elderly people have definite therapeutic implications for the resolution of pathological conditions. The aging person exhibits progressively limited thermoregulation, skin integrity, membrane permeability, lung capacity, cardiac reserve, organ function, nervous system adaptability, muscle flexibility, metabolism, and sensory acuity. Nurses research the extent to which the decremental physiological health of the elderly can be stabilized or improved by changes in nursing practices (see Tables 4.5 to 4.11).

Food and Fluid Intake, Oral Hygiene

The fluid intake of the elderly in nursing homes is of particular concern to nurses (see Table 4.5). Three studies documented that fluid intake was significantly higher for noninstitutionalized elderly. As the age of the nursing home resident increased, the adequate intake of water decreased. Semidependent residents had a higher risk of inadequate fluid intake than did dependent or independent residents. The researchers recommended that fluid intake be used as a quality of care indicator in nursing home audits.

The results of nutritional assessments in hospital settings were described in three studies. One identified that patients on enteral feedings were malnourished at the initiation of this method, and no improvement in caloric intake occurred over a period of time. Common problems were aspiration (26.4%) and diarrhea (60.3%). In a second study, an extended care facility introduced a dietary supplement program following several audits in which substandard food intake was documented.

Methods for administering tube feedings have also been researched. Small bore tubes and moderate temperatures for feedings were preferred, with small bore tubes increasing the feasibility of tube feeding patients at home. Research has demonstrated that oral hygiene for nursing home residents implemented every four hours statistically improved salivation, condition of the membranes, and lip moisture.

Nocturnal Behavior

Nursing research on sleep patterns of hospitalized elderly, nonhospitalized elderly, and nursing home residents indicated that pattern variations were individual, although after age 85 there is a significant increase in sleep latency and total sleep time (see Table 4.6). Other sleep studies were discussed earlier in this paper. The overuse of neuroleptic medications indicates the need for more research and changes in clinical practice, especially since these medications increase disorientation and risk of falls.

Incontinence

Untreated, uncontrolled incontinence is a frequently stated reason for admission to long-term care facilities. Nurses have researched methods of incontinence assessment, padding methods, toileting procedures, bladder training programs, and psychological stress caused by incontinence (see Table 4.7).

Unfortunately, toileting programs to control incontinence have been demonstrated to be labor-intensive and not as cost-efficient as barrier pads. External urinary devices are an acceptable alternative to indwelling catheters when bladder training will not work. However, external devices also may contribute to increased risk of infection and skin damage. Several studies explored the use of behavior modification to alter incontinence. In one study of 60 elderly people who were at risk of being incontinent and 14 who were urinary incontinent, self-care education and treatment resulted in six regaining continence and none becoming incontinent.

A similar study resulted in 79% of 14 incontinent patients becoming continent.

Pressure Sores

The topic of skin integrity and pressure sores is among the most frequently researched areas. The 16 studies presented indicate the interest of researchers in this area (see Table 4.8). Highly reliable at-risk assessment tools have been developed. Infratherapy has been found to be cost-effective for small sores, and a second study indicated that a specialized bed also was effective. The use of a programmed plan of care developed by nurses reduced the incidence of pressure sores from 12% to 2% in a 360-bed skilled nursing facility. Water mattresses, air fluidized beds, small weight shifts, and repositioning are other pressure sore therapies that have been researched by nurses.

Both the prevention and treatment of pressure sores are expensive. Nurses spend a great deal of time turning patients. Preventive equipment can cost up to $185 a day. The Braden scale, which has been extensively tested, is used by nurses to select those patients at risk and focus preventive measures on them, thereby eliminating wasted time and resources on those who do not need it. The National Institutes of Health's Center for Nursing Research has awarded a three-year grant to conduct a multisite study of pressure sore risk.

Thermoregulation and Cardiovascular Parameters

The decremental changes of aging increased the risk of hypothermia for the elderly. Ten nursing studies of temperature regulation, conducted across settings, lead to the following conclusions:

- extra head and body coverage during surgery decreases risks accompanying thermal stress;
- oxygen therapy does not significantly affect oral temperatures;
- the normal body temperature of people ages 60 to 94 ranges nearly 3°; and
- temperature variability increases with age (see Table 4.9).

Mean body temperatures of the elderly are below adult norms, substantiating the extent to which the elderly are at risk of hypothermia. Seven nursing studies used physiological parameters to substantiate how to position and obtain the most accurate status readings for cardiac patients and critically ill patients (see Table 4.9).

Exercise

Ten nursing studies suggested that exercise not only improves the strength, flexibility, balance, and cardiac reserve of elderly persons, but also has a positive relationship to self-esteem and self-perceived good health (see Table 4.10). Additionally, exercise exhibited an inverse relationship to depression.

One study of patients with rheumatoid arthritis concluded that nonweight-bearing, active range-of-motion exercises performed in the evening reduced stiffness and increased mobility more effectively than morning exercises alone. In a limited study of a four-week exercise program for 19 institutionalized elderly, independent self-care ability was unaffected, suggesting further study. One nurse researcher suggested that regular outdoor walking be instituted for all ambulatory nursing home residents, even those using canes and walkers, after a test comparison of this population with a retirement village population.

Foot Care

Foot care is an often ignored area of elderly care. Lack of foot care can lead to infection, loss of mobility, and amputation. Five scientific studies indicated prevalence of untreated dry skin and foot problems in the elderly and identified nursing therapies that are effective (see Table 4.11). Nurse-managed foot clinics in community centers have demonstrated cost-effectiveness through early detection and referral of debilitation problems, especially for elderly diabetic patients.

Cognitive Function

Cognitive function includes all thought and reasoning processes, such as problem solving, perception, memory, and judgment. The ability of the elderly to comprehend and learn health education is a research concern of nurses.

Health Teaching Needs

Findings from three studies validated that the elderly can learn (see Table 4.12). In one study, 10% of the elderly participants felt they were too old to learn, despite clear evidence that age does not affect intelligence, and that self-paced study is advantageous. A meta-analysis of 68 studies of surgical patients who received preoperative instruction

supports the positive effect of teaching on operative outcomes. Three studies assessed the knowledge and behavior
relationships of lens implant patients, hypertensive patients,
and women practicing self-examination of their breasts.

Confusion

Cognitive dysfunction is a common symptom presented
in conjunction with cardiovascular diseases, metabolic disorders, hematological disorders, and overmedication (see
Table 4.13). Five research studies on confused states of
elderly patients documented the prevalence of cognitive
dysfunction in health care settings.

One study of 60 hospitalized elderly identified that 38%
developed confusion within six days of admission. In a study
of hospitalized versus institutionalized elderly, environmental deficits contributed to cognitive disturbances in the institutionalized. In a similar study, acute postoperative
confusion was effectively reduced through additional
patient orientation and clarification, as well as through cor-
rection of patients' sensory deficits and staff education.
Another study documented that over one-half of elderly
people who were hospitalized for hip fractures evidenced
postoperative confusion despite the fact that no previous
history of cognitive impairment existed.

Confusion in the elderly leads to a high incidence of falls,
agitation, and injury to self and others. Nurse researchers
are examining each facet of behavior precursors of confusion. Tools are being developed to predict confusion and
aggressive behavior episodes. For instance, data suggest
that the placement of a mentally incompetent skilled nursing home resident with a mentally competent person results
in a decline in the mental and emotional status of the latter.
In a random sample of 1,139 patients in 42 skilled nursing
home facilities, it was found that 64.2% had significant
behavioral problems. A pharmacological approach to the
problem of confusion and aggressive behavior is inadequate
in many cases and inhumane in others.

The National Institutes of Health's Center for Nursing
Research recently awarded a five-year grant to continue
investigations of the problem of acute confusion among
hospitalized patients. The ultimate goal is to show that
assessment and pattern-specific interventions (i.e., in cases
of confusion related to toxic metabolic responses, physiological instability, and environmental changes) are more
effective than usual interventions, and that nursing care
reduces the incidence of confusion and improves function

among hospitalized patients.

Humane measures to reduce agitated and aggressive behavior of mentally incompetent hospital and nursing home patients are labor-intensive and inadequately covered by current professional staffing ratios. In a sample of patients ages 75 and older on a hospital medical ward, almost all required bathing assistance, 40% experienced incontinence, 37% were disoriented, 30% were confused, 14% were agitated or aggressive, 25% had visual or hearing deficits, and 19% required physical restraints. Current reimbursement formulas do not take into account the time required to care for people with these deficits.

Psychosocial Health Dysfunction

The belief that old age is a period of tranquility and contemplation is a myth. Research findings support the facts that older people experience more stress due to the infirmities of aging and have less adequate coping mechanisms than the non-elderly. Nurses identify and maximize the coping strategies of the elderly, and offer education and adaptation support.

Bereavement

Thirteen studies focused on the psychosocial health dysfunctions and coping resources of bereaved widows and widowers, in order to effectively help them adjust to their loss (see Table 4.14). Effective coping resources included social support, strong religious beliefs, rituals, and belief in control over bereavement. Good prior mental health related positively to less psychosocial or physical dysfunction. *Less* helpful coping strategies included overt anger; self-blame; increased sleeping; use of fantasy; avoidance of people; and taking antidepressants, tranquilizers, sedatives, and alcoholic beverages. Bereavement, contrary to commonly held notions, was not related to problem drinking.

Whether divorced or widowed, an individual's positive perception of personal health was the major indicator of subjective well-being. A grief resolution index can reliably identify persons who continue to experience bereavement distress.

Relocation

Psychosocial dysfunction related to relocation or institutionalization is another health problem of legitimate concern to nursing. Ten studies described the risk factors associated with relocation events (see Table 4.15).

One study delineated four nursing home admission adjustment phases: disorganization (four to six weeks), reorganization (six to 12 weeks), relationship building (three months), and stabilization (after three months). Residents tended to return to the disorganization phase when crises occurred. Anger or anxiety before relocation increased the risk of death following relocation. Other physical risk factors associated with relocation included fever, pneumonia, upper respiratory infection, urinary tract infection, and hospital admission. A loss of identity and sense of self accompanied the decrease in personal possessions. Research indicated that successful relocation is predicated on reasonable preparation.

Issues Surrounding Quality of Death/End-of-Life Directives

Advances in technology have created sophisticated life-extension modalities. In reality, the same modalities that save lives are often used to extend death. Influenced by the "death phobia" of Western culture, many elderly suffer painful and extremely costly deaths.

Research in this area is just beginning to surface, and it is crucial in identifying indicators of quality of health for older people. As the Rubenstein, Rubenstein, and Josephson paper points out, quality of death—along with quality of life—must be addressed in planning for our future health care system.

Research in the literature clearly indicates that consumers and health care professionals strongly believe that individuals and their families should be involved in planning end-of-life directives (see Table 4.16). The research is also clear on the fact that patients are rarely included in this kind of planning; very few institutions even broach this subject when patients are admitted. Researchers in one study surveyed patients about their end-of-life directives upon admission to the hospital for elective surgery. They also studied patients' responses to participating in this survey. The overwhelming majority of patients were supportive of such a process and wanted their physicians informed. 15% of the patients, however, did indicate an increase in anxiety.

Research has found that most individuals have strong feelings about end-of-life directives, yet have rarely discussed this with their physicians or nurses. Billions of dollars are spent every year on extension of death—80% of individuals now die in institutions. Financially and ethically, this topic needs research and policy if this nation is to adequately prepare for 21st century health care.

Family-Focused Issues

Elderly people and their families turn to health care professionals for support and technical knowledge when they can no longer manage the dependency crises and disease management of old age. It is through task sharing between health care providers and families or significant others that the health and well-being of the frail elderly are most sustained or improved. The underlying goals of this shared support system are to fulfill three needs: socialization, carrying out the tasks of daily living, and personal assistance during health crises. Nurses have researched family members' needs and responses, as well as the effectiveness of nursing support for these caregivers.

Family Caregiver Issues

Six descriptive studies examined the multiple factors which influence the quality of family caregiving for the frail elderly (see Table 4.17). In one of these studies, 22 multigenerational households were reviewed, concluding that one of the most pervasive problems is lack of communication between generations. In another study of 39 health providers, a decision model was developed for identifying and intervening in cases of suspected elder abuse and neglect.

Fourteen studies described the stressful effects of caregiving in general and in specific situations where the elderly family member has dementia or chronic obstructive pulmonary disease (see Table 4.17). Nursing measures found to reduce stress included easing families' fears, interpreting caregiver/family member interactions, social skill training, and assisting couples to resolve care problems through communication. One study found no significant decrease in reported stress for caregivers in group therapy.

Nursing Home Placement Decision Criteria

Nine studies addressed how nursing home placement decisions are made by family caregivers (see Table 4.18). Evidence suggested that in situations where the elderly family member is demented, family stress is a better predictor of nursing home placement than is the severity of the dementia. Two studies substantiated that a common pattern for nursing home admissions is a physical illness requiring hospitalization, followed by a physician advising nursing home placement. One study found that fewer than 50% of the residents decided on their own nursing home admissions. Difficulty in ambulation and confusion were the most common problems precipitating admissions.

Three publications described pilot projects in which supportive home care services had proven very beneficial for caregivers. Positive patient outcomes identified in these home care projects included increased capabilities in activities of daily living and increased mobility compared to similar nursing home patients. A fourth pilot project, a block nursing program, studied the effectiveness of case management by public health nurses living in the neighborhood. The program succeeded in keeping dependent elderly persons in their homes at low costs, while meeting high care standards. Three research strategies for assessing the health of elderly persons in urban neighborhoods included surveys, census track data, and ethnography.

Nursing Staff Issues

Nurses and nursing assistants are the primary caregivers in long-term care facilities. The Institute of Medicine's *Report Improving the Quality of Care in Nursing Homes* (Committee on Nursing Home Regulation, 1986) stated that one of the major factors affecting the quality of care and the quality of life in nursing homes is the number and quality of the nursing staff. These same conclusions and concerns apply to care of the elderly in acute care, home, and ambulatory settings. When assessing the quality of care for the elderly, the competency of the nursing staff and their effect on patient processes and outcomes are major indicators. The studies in this section are indicative of the nursing research being conducted to validate this relationship (see Table 4.19).

One meta-analysis reviewed 84 studies of 4,146 subjects to test the effect of nursing practices based on experimental, controlled research over an eight-year period. The investigators concluded that patients who received research-based nursing interventions could expect 28% better outcomes than 72% of the patients in control groups who received standard nursing care.

Four studies addressed the effect of staff competency on patient outcomes. In one pretest and posttest study, professional nurses participated in a training program on how to conduct cognitive group therapy and applied the techniques with 46 depressed elderly patients in community health settings. The patients displayed significant improvement compared to depressed elderly cared for by personnel without special training. A review of 200 incidents of violent behavior indicated that the incidents occurred because of insufficient staffing and the predominance of unskilled personnel. A related nursing home study documented that there was no relationship between knowledge of the nursing staff about confusion in the elderly and years of nursing experience. Education updates on dementia, management of reversible confusion, and altered physiological states were recommended. In hospitals, a decentralized nursing care environment was credited with reducing confusion in disturbed elderly.

In a comparison study of four skilled nursing facilities, researchers determined that the quality of care, as assessed by the Quality Patient Care Scale (QualPacs) tool, varied according to the number and skill level of personnel. Care improves when the ratio of professional nursing personnel to nonlicensed personnel is high.

Even when nursing competency is present, poor nurse utilization or insufficient numbers of personnel reduce the quantity and quality of nursing care available to the patient. A Veterans Administration work sampling study conducted over two weeks in a 1,600-bed facility concluded that 657 hours of nursing time was devoted to non-nursing clerical functions—affecting medication administration and supportive care. Productive clinical care time by nurses involved in home care decreased as paperwork time increased. In one study of home care nurses, time spent in the offices documenting new Medicare forms increased from 19% to 28%.

In a study of 1,000 males admitted to nursing homes after hospitalization, the outcomes of decreased mortality, health status improvement, and eventual discharge were found to be positively related to the ratio of registered nurse hours per patient. Two studies indicated that when nursing care patients were assigned a primary nurse who was totally accountable for their care, incidents of pressure sores decreased 75%, mortality decreased 18%, overall care and family satisfaction increased, and turnover in nursing staff decreased 29%.

Nine studies validated that behaviors of staff affect patient outcomes. Patients perceived that nurses on a coronary care unit who assessed their status and gave physical care were more caring than nurses who taught or conducted delegated medical tasks.

In one nursing home, attending behaviors significantly increased residents' mental status. A related study demonstrated that touch combined with verbal requests was more effective than the request alone when caring for elderly confused patients. Patient satisfaction increased when the nurse and patient set mutually agreed upon health outcomes and when patients were asked if they needed assistance. Patients valued interpersonal aspects of care above "hotel services." Nursing home patients who could identify specific nurses as confidantes tested highest on life-satisfaction scores. A work sampling study of 400 nursing employees in a long-term care facility indicated nursing personnel communicated with the residents during 80%-90% of the care activities they conducted.

Two studies of the attitudes of nursing home personnel toward aging and the aged revealed that skilled nursing personnel were not as negative toward aging as originally perceived. Registered nurses had more positive attitudes than licensed practical nurses and nursing assistants. Licensed practical nurses were the least positive.

Preliminary findings from a current investigation at the University of Wisconsin-Milwaukee suggest that a) the level of education of the charge nurse relates positively to residents' satisfaction with the nursing home, and b) high turnover of registered nurses and nursing assistants relates negatively to residents' life-satisfaction.

Retention of nurses qualified for long-term care is a concern. Geriatric nurse practitioners identify primary care assignments and patient appreciation as the two factors most effective in attracting and retaining competent nurses who specialize in long-term care. When 46 nursing home administrators were surveyed about the effectiveness of nurse practitioners in quality improvement and cost containment, their responses were "overwhelmingly positive in both regards."   □

Table 4.1
TECHNICAL QUALITY OF CARE: QUALITY OF LIFE, LIFE SATISFACTION, AND HEALTH PROMOTION (Selected References)

Reference	Study Population	Design	Findings
Laborde & Powers (1985)	N = 160 osteoarthritic subjects; 2 ambulatory care settings & 2 hospitals	Correlational study examining relationships between life satisfaction & illness symptoms	Life satisfaction related to less pain, perception of health, & internal control
Hoeffer (1987)	N = 816	Secondary analysis of national survey of aged, examining personal and social factors on outlook on quality of life (QOL)	Never-married women were more educated, less lonely, & healthier than widows; health & loneliness best predictors of QOL
McDaniel (1987)	N = 91 random sample	Descriptive correlational study to test relationships of QOL, perceived health, & other variables	Health promotion behaviors best predictor of QOL
Foster (1987)	N = 100 blacks, ages 60-89, Southwestern USA	Descriptive design of life satisfaction, health promotion, exercise, & self actualization	Current health significantly correlated with life satisfaction
Walker, Volken, Schrist, & Pender (1988)	N = 452	Comparative study of middle-aged and young persons on health promoting behaviors	Older adults scored highest on health promotion; exercise lowest score of groups
Pohl & Fuller (1980)	N = 50 residents in long-term care facilities	Hierarchical multiple regression to examine predictors of morale related to relocation	Decisional control & social interaction strongest influences on morale
Ryden (1984)	N = 113 patients from 4 randomly selected long-term care facilities (urban-proprietary)	Descriptive correlational	Perception of control highest predictor of morale; functional dependency, health, & socioeconomic status (SES) affected morale for intermediate patients
Maglivy (1985)	N = 66 hearing-impaired females	Path analysis to determine predictors of QOL	Best predictors of QOL: perceived health, functional social support, & social hearing handicap
Bowsher (1987)	N = 67 cognitively intact elderly from 6 long-term care facilities	Descriptive study of variance related to psychological well-being	Control expectancy, self-rated health, and perceived constraint of situation explain significant amounts of variance

Other selected references in this area: (Brown & McCreedy, 1986; Cassels, 1988; Chang, 1978; Chang, Uman, Linn, Ware, & Kane, 1985; Dean, 1988; Devey, 1990; Dolinsky, 1987; Ferrans, Powers, & Kasch, 1987; Flynn, 1986; Flynn & Frantz, 1987; Folden, 1990; Forsyth, Delaney, & Gresham, 1984; Frank-Stromberg, 1988; Fuller & Larson, 1980; Gilson & Coates, 1980; Hargrove-Huttle, 1989; Horgan, 1987; Johnson, Cloyd, & Wer, 1982; Johnson, 1987; Johnson, Foxall, Kidwell-Udin, Miller, & Stolzer, 1984; Keller, Levinthal, Prohaska, & Levinthal, 1989; King, Figge, & Harman, 1986; Lacey, 1989; Mills, 1986; O'Connel, Hamera, Kanapp, Cassmeyer, Eaks, & Fox, 1984; Oudt, 1989; Padilla & Grant, 1985; Pascucci, 1988; Rauckhorst, 1987; Ryden, 1985; Schafer, 1989; Schank & Lough, 1989; Schwartz, 1980; Schwirian, 1982; Sellers, 1986; Simon, 1990; Speake, Cowart, & Pellet, 1989; Spitzer, Dobson, Hall, Chesterman, Levi, & Shepard, 1981; Steinke, 1988; Terpstra, Terpestra, Plawecki, & Streeter, 1989; Thomas, 1988; Thomas & Hooper, 1983; Trice, 1986; Trippet, 1989)

Table 4.2
TECHNICAL QUALITY OF CARE: MENTAL HEALTH OF OLDER PEOPLE (Selected References)

Reference	Study Population	Design	Findings
Reed (1986)	N = 114, 57 terminally ill & 57 non-terminally ill	Descriptive design of 2 matched groups; examining well-being & religiousness	Supports developmental view of terminal illness; terminal illness more religious; positive relationship between religiousness & well-being
Reed (1986)	N = 56 elderly, 28 depressed & 28 mentally healthy, matched groups	Time series longitudinal design, 2-group comparison	Depressed group had significantly lower developmental scores for 3 time periods; in nondepressed group, developmental resources influenced health—reversed with depressed; implications for intervention with depression
Burckhardt (1987)	N = 41 controlled research studies on effects of nursing intervention	Meta-analysis	Mean outcome of treatment group was significantly higher than mean outcome of control group; improved from 50% to 70%; nursing effective in enhancing mental health of aged
Braun (1987)	N = 53 women in long-term care facility; 28 failure to thrive & 25 nonfailure	Time series longitudinal design, 2-group comparison	Failure to thrive, physically & cognitively disabled, more depressed; both groups consumed inadequate calories, calcium, & folic acid
Fishman (1989)	N = 115 men & women, ages 65-93	Correlational design to study relationship between death anxiety, life review, & ego integrity	Death anxiety was significantly correlated (negatively) with ego integrity & life review; the higher the QOL review, the lower the death anxiety

Other selected references in this area: (Cassels, Fortinash, & Eckstein, 1981; Christian, Dluhy, O'Neill, 1989; Christman, McConnell, Pfeiffer, Webster, Schmitt, & Ries, 1988; Collins, 1988; Daily & Futrell, 1989; Dietx, 1986; Farran & McCann, 1989; Farran & Popovich, 1990; Farran, Salloway, & Clark, 1990; Greene & Monahan, 1982; Hoeffer, 1987; Keane & Sells, 1990; Leja, 1989; Louis, 1981; Nelson, 1990; Nelson, 1989; Newman & Gaudino, 1984; Powers, 1988; Poznanski, 1987; Preston & Dellasega, 1990; Rainwater, 1988; Reed, 1989; Rodgers, 1989; Scott, Oberst, & Bookbinder, 1984; Slimmer, Edwards-Beckett, LeSage, Ellor, & Lopez, 1990; Slimmer, Lopez, LeSage, & Ellor, 1987; Wright, 1990; Zucker, 1987)

Table 4.3
TECHNICAL QUALITY OF CARE: RELAXATION & MULTIMETHOD NURSING (Selected References)

Reference	Study Population	Design	Findings
DeMoss (1980)	N = 400 individual chemotherapy treatments, 70 clients, majority 60 years of age	Quasi-experimental design to test nursing intervention	Nausea & vomiting rarely present; program enabled clients to continue chemotherapy as long as possible with very few side effects
Dixon (1984)	N = 88 patients randomly assigned to 1 of 4 treatment groups; nutritionally at-risk cancer patients, mean age 59.6 years	Repeated measures experimental design, 4 groups: relaxation, nutritional support, both, & neither; dependent variable: weight & muscle circumference	Relaxation group had most significant weight gain or maintenance; greatest loss was found in control group
Frank (1985)	N = 15 cancer patients using antiemetics; retested after including music & visual imagery	Quasi-experimental pre-test and posttest design to test nursing intervention	Perceived degree of vomiting & anxiety both significantly reduced with music and imagery
Kutlenios (1985)	N = 45 subjects ages 60 & over, recruited from community residential complexes	Nonequivalent group quasi-experimental design to assess differences between holistic treatment, mental health treatment, physical treatment, & control	Holistic intervention achieved highest score with increased internal control, although significance not reached
Fakouri & Jones (1987)	N = 18, mean age 73	Quasi-experimental design to test slow-stroke back rub	Effective intervention as measured by physiologic indicators

Other selected references in this area: (Hamilton, 1989; Rice, Caldwell, Butler, & Robinson, 1986; Zimmerman, Pozehl, Duncan, & Schmitz, 1989)

Table 4.4
TECHNICAL QUALITY OF CARE: SELF-CARE & ACTIVITIES OF DAILY LIVING (Selected References)

Reference	Study Population	Design	Findings
Lambert (1985)	N = 92 women, mean age 55, arthritic	Descriptive correlational design to assess factors associated with well-being & other variables	Positive correlations between dependence on others & length of illness; pain & difficulty with ADL significantly correlated with well-being (negatively)
Lewis, Kane, Kretin, & Clark (1985)	N = 563 patients discharged from 24 long-term care facilities	Retrospective descriptive study to identify outcomes	Only 28% were discharged to home; ADL scores were only variable that predicted survival in immediate and 2-year follow-up; social support predicted immediate survival only
Colling (1985)	N = 118 randomly selected from 70 long-term care facilities	Casual modeling correlational survey	Control over ADL significantly correlated with well-being; control over ADL significantly associated with nursing staff support; age & functional status influence well-being
Mahoney (1985)	N = 22 previously able-bodied subjects with unilateral stroke	Quasi-experimental explanatory model addressing interplay of variables, versus traditional model based on physical predictors alone	Multidimensional model explained 39% of variance; physical model explained 13%; physical model may not be sensitive to self-care, which strongly influences institutionalization rate and QOL
Kelly-Hayes (1987)	N = 82, 41 stroke & 41 nonstroke	Retrospective correlational study using Framingham data	Stroke patients 4 times more depressed; dependence in ADL best predictor of institutionalization; patients physically impaired also cognitively impaired

Other selected references in this area: (Buckwalter, Cusack, Stidles, Wadle, & Beaver, 1989; Davidson & Young, 1985; DeVon & Powers, 1984; Hain & Chen, 1986; Harrell, McConnell, Wildman, & Samsa, 1989; Hess, 1986; Johnson & Moore, 1988; Karl, 1982; King, Norsen, Robertson, & Hicks, 1987; Labi, Phillips, & Gresham, 1980; Lantz, 1985; Magilvy, Brown, & Dydyn, 1988; Mion, Frengley, & Adams, 1986; Patsdaughter & Pesznecker, 1988; Pensiero & Adams, 1987; Shamanasky & Hamilton, 1979)

Table 4.5
TECHNICAL QUALITY OF CARE: FOOD & FLUID INTAKE, ORAL HYGIENE (Selected References)

Reference	Study Population	Design	Findings
Meyer (1987)	N = 67 elderly residents of 2 long-term care facilities	Nonparticipant observation study, recording of fluid intake	Only 3 subjects met intake requirements; mean adequacy 76.6%; those who had higher intake were younger, male, & independent of experiencing speech or vision impairment.
Adams (1988)	N = 60, 30 institutionalized & 30 noninstitutionalized; ages 65-85; exclusion of cognitive impairments, major disability, & diabetes	2-group correlational design	Institutionalized elderly had significantly less intake (2115 cc vs. 1570 cc); intake for institutionalized elderly occurred at medication time or meal time, indicating dependence on nursing staff.
Brown & Stegman (1988)	N = 94 randomly selected acute care patients	Instrument validation to assess sensitivity & specificity of nutritonal risk	Sensitivity = 95%; specificity = 89%; cost-effective screening device to identify patients at nutritional risk
Pritchard (1988)	N = 20 patients with respiratory tract infections on tube feedings	Retrospective design to ascertain differences in feeding tubes as related to infection	70% of gastric feeding tubes with infection was related to large bore Levine type tube; small bore weighted tube recommended

Other selected references in this area: (Athlin, Norberg, Axelsson, Moller, & Nordstrom, 1989; Cagawa-Busby, Heltkempr, Hansen, Hanson, & Vanderburg, 1988; Collinsworth & Boyle, 1989; DeWalt, 1975; Eaton, Mitchell-Bonair, & Friedman, 1986; Flynn, Norton, & Fisher, 1987; Gasper, 1988; Howe, Coulton, Almon, & Sandrick, 1980; Longman & DeWalt, 1986; Michaelsson, Norberg, & Norberg, 1987; Spitzer, 1988)

Table 4.6
TECHNICAL QUALITY OF CARE: NOCTURNAL BEHAVIOR (Selected References)

Reference	Study Population	Design	Findings
Pacini & Fitzpatrick (1982)	N = 38, ages 60-82, 16 hospitalized & 16 nonhospitalized	Descriptive design to examine sleep pattern differences, 2-group design	Significant differences between nocturnal sleep, other sleep, bedtime sleep, & awakenings
Hayter (1983)	N = 212 random healthy noninstitutionalized, ages 60-82	Descriptive study, sleep among different age groups of elderly via sleep charts & surveys	Significant increase in time in bed, total sleep time, number of naps, & amount of wake time after sleep onset in those over age 75

Other selected references in this area: (Clapin-French, 1986; Gress, Hassanein, & Bahr, 1981; Young, Muir-Nash, & Ninos, 1988)

Table 4.7
TECHNICAL QUALITY OF CARE: INCONTINENCE (Selected References)

Reference	Study Population	Design	Findings
Pritchard (1985)	N = 34 elderly residents who developed urinary incontinence	Retrospective epidemio-logical approach to identify factors associated with outbreak of infections	External urinary devices were contributing to infec-tions; may present greater risk than previously expected; adult incontinence barrier pads may provide greater safety
Pearson & Droessler (1988)	N = 96 elders living in room & board facility with small infirmary available; 74 com-pleted study at 6 months	Quasi-experimental design testing treatment groups with 60 at-risk patients; 14 incon-tinent; treatment & nursing intervention to support self-care	6 regained continence; no new incontinence
Yu, Kaltreider, Hu, Igou, & Craighead (1989)	N = 96 female residents of 7 long-term care facilities; mean age 85.3	Descriptive study to examine instrument validity & assess symptoms associated with incontinence	Those with incontinence show depressive symptoms & feelings of shame
Baigis-Smith, Jakobac-Smith, Rose, & Newman (1989)	N = 54 cognitively intact patients with stress or complex types of incontinence	Quasi-experimental pre-test and posttest group, repeated measures, 2-year project; treatment & nursing inter-vention, including Kegel, relaxation, biofeedback, & habit training	Significant decrease in urinary accidents per week; maintained at 6 month and 1 year follow-up

Other selected references in this area: (Barker & Mitteness, 1989; Brink, Sampselle, Wells, Diokno, & Gillis, 1989; Burgio, Jones, & Engel, 1988; Diokno, Wells, & Brink, 1987; Grant, 1982; Gross, 1990; Haeker, 1985; Hu, Kaltreider, & Igou, 1990; Hu, Kaltreider, & Igou, 1989; Kaltreider, Hu, Igou, Yu, & Craighead, 1990; Lara, Troup, & Beadleson-Baird, 1990; LeSage, Slimmer, Lopez, Ellor, 1989; Long, 1985; Miller, 1990; Oberst, Graham, Geller, Maus, Stearns, & Tiernan, 1981; Ouslander, Marishita, Balustein, Orzeck, Dunn, & Sayre, 1987; Robb, 1985; Schneille, Traughber, Morgan, Embry, Binion, & Coleman, 1983; Simons, 1985; Sowell, Schneille, Hu, & Traughber, 1987; Wells, Brink, & Diokono, 1987; Whitman & Kursh, 1987; Yu, 1987; Yu & Kaltreider, 1987)

Table 4.8
TECHNICAL QUALITY OF CARE: PRESSURE SORES (Selected References)

Reference	Study Population	Design	Findings
Droessler & Maibusch (1982)	360-bed skilled nursing facility, ages 60-102	1-year descriptive study examining decubiti incidence & response to nursing program plan of care	Incidence of decubiti decreased from 12% to 2%
Frantz & Kinney (1986)	N = 76, ages 65-97, mean age 80	Correlational study to examine relationship between sebum secretion & occurrence of dry skin	Findings refute belief that decreased sebaceous activity is responsible for skin dryness; relationship exists between skin dryness & age
Allman, Walker, Hart, Laprade, Knoll, & Smith (1987)	N = 140 randomized clinical trial, 65 completing study; patients hospitalized with pressure sores	Quasi-experimental, 2 groups; air fluid & conventional treatment with foam mattress	Air-fluidized beds more effective, especially for large pressure sores
Bergstrom, Braden, Laguzza, & Holman (1987)	Secondary analysis of 3 studies, N = 50-54, mean ages 75-79	Psychometric analysis of instrument to predict pressure sore risk	The Braden Scale was found highly reliable when used by RNs; .99 specificity 64-90%

Other selected references in this area: (Becker & Goodemote, 1984; Black, VanBerkel, Green, Everett, & Krilyk, 1987; Blom, 1985; Bristow, Goldfarb, & Green, 1987; Brown, Boosinger, Black, & Gaspar, 1985; Clarke, 1988; Diekmann, 1984; Distel, 1981; Hyland & Kirkland, 1980; Munro, Brown, & Heitman, 1989; Pajk, Craven, Cameron, Shipps, & Bennum, 1986; Reynolds, 1989; Stoneberg, Pitcook, & Myton, 1986; Wirtz, 1987)

Table 4.9
TECHNICAL QUALITY OF CARE: THERMOREGULATION AND CARDIOVASCULAR PARAMETERS
(Selected References)

Reference	Study Population	Design	Findings
Higgins (1983)	N = 60 well elderly, 65-90 years	Descriptive, exploratory study of normal temperature of well-elderly	Average temperature for sample was 97.9; 98.1 for females; 97.9 for males; temperatures were found to decrease & variability increase with increasing age
Biddle & Biddle (1985)	N = 127 elderly patients ages 65-90, undergoing abdominal surgery	Experimental design; testing impact of using head covering during surgery	Wearing nonhazardous head covering significantly decreased risk of hypothermia for elders
Folta, Storm, & Therrien (1987)	N = 149, divided into 2 age groups: below 55 & above 55; healthy adults, mean age 64 for older group	Experimental 2-group design to examine effect of Valsalva on blood pressure and heart rate in 2 age groups	Compensatory mechanisms that regulate blood pressure & heart rate during Valsalva less effective in healthy older than healthy younger
Banasik & Steadman (1987)	N = 60 patients, mean age 62, admitted for coronary revascularization	Quasi-experimental Pa02 levels related to position	Pa02 level is higher in right lateral and supine positions in postoperative coronary bypass patients; left lateral associated with lower Pa02 levels, especially when left atelectasis is present

Other selected references in this area: (Davis & Lentz, 1989; Doering & Dracup, 1988; Dressler, Smejkal, & Ruffolo, 1983; Durham, Swanson, & Pulford, 1986; Folta, Metzger, & Therrien, 1989; Heidenreich & Giuffre, 1990; Kolanowski & Gunter, 1981; Mason, 1987; Polyneaux, Papciak, & Woem, 1987; Schneider, 1987; Storm, Metzger, & Therrien, 1989; Thatcher, 1983; White, Thurston, Blackmore, Green, & Hannah, 1987; Wirtz, 1987)

Table 4.10
TECHNICAL QUALITY OF CARE: EXERCISE (Selected References)

Reference	Study Population	Design	Findings
Parent & Wahll (1984)	N = 30 residents of a senior center, ages 60 and over	Correlational design comparing those with hobbies of various physical exertion to those with no hobbies	Subjects involved in hobbies were less depressed than subjects who were not involved; hobbies requiring more physical exertion had positive relationship to self-esteem and inverse relationship to depression
Byers (1985)	N = 30 patients from outpatient rheumatoid arthritis clinic; mean age 61.9	Quasi-experimental 2-group comparison of morning exercise or morning & evening exercise.	Elastic stiffness & subjective ratings of stiffness were less and mobility was greater when evening exercises performed
Magnani (1986)	N = 110 healthy non-institutionalized elderly, ages 60-90	Survey design to compare levels of hardiness, self-perceived health, & physical activity	Higher levels of hardiness & self-perceived health had higher levels of activity
Gueldner & Spradley (1988)	N = 64, 32 in each group of elderly residents	Quasi-experimental design to test effects of regular outdoor walking	Results indicate that regular outdoor walking should be instituted as quality care for all long-term care residents, even if assistance of walkers or canes necessary

Other selected references in this area: (Basset, McClamrock, & Schmelzer, 1982; Clough & Maurin, 1983; Colanowski & Gunter, 1988; Karl, 1982; Melillo, 1980; Roberts, 1989)

Table 4.11
TECHNICAL QUALITY OF CARE: FOOT CARE (Selected References)

Reference	Study Population	Design	Findings
Schank & Conrad (1977)	N = 125 well-elderly, community residents	Descriptive survey design	89% of the women & 61% of the men reported foot problems; foot soaks most common treatment used
Brown, Boosinger, Black, Gaspar, & Sather (1982)	N = 31 elderly in a long-term care facility	Descriptive design to analyze outcomes from nursing innovation	After innovation there was a decrease in skin dryness & softening of callouses at immediate & 4-month follow-up
Haviland & Garlinghouse (1985)	N = 160 initial visits; 256 follow-up visits at college of nursing foot clinic	Descriptive retrospective design to analyze costs & outcomes	Decreased costs resulted, as well as increase of early detection & prevention

Other selected references in this area: (Chung, 1983; Frantz & Kinney, 1986)

Table 4.12
TECHNICAL QUALITY OF CARE: HEALTH TEACHING NEEDS (Selected References)

Reference	Study Population	Design	Findings
Baldini (1981)	N = 45 elderly in community with hypertension, ages 65-90, mean age 77	Descriptive design; explore general knowledge of hypertensives	Participants had insufficient knowledge related to hypertension; also little evidence that they had been informed about their disease
Hathaway (1986)	68 studies; 2413 experimental subjects & 1605 control subjects	Meta-analysis of pre-operative instruction	Average patient who received pre-operative instruction at 66% of a similar group without pre-operative instruction; all categories of studies had positive effects
Kim (1986)	N = 105 randomly selected elderly assigned to 3 groups of education	Quasi-experimental design to compare fast-paced, slow-paced, and self-paced health care learning	Learning performances under fast-paced and slow-paced conditions did not differ; self-paced was superior to both other conditions
Craig (1988)	N = 55 men from Veterans Administration centers in Southeast USA with diagnosis of hypertension, ages 55 and older	Descriptive study with multiple regression to identify characteristics of older men & their ability to comprehend health education material	Reliable predictors of ability to comprehend included achieved grade level, current grade level, readability of material, race, & choice of materials

Other selected references in this area: (Bahr & Griss, 1982; Check & Wurzbach, 1984; DeBlase, Badziong, & Jones, 1988; Lashley, 1987; Shamanasky & Hamilton, 1979)

Table 4.13
TECHNICAL QUALITY OF CARE: CONFUSION (Selected References)

Reference	Study Population	Design	Findings
Wiltzius, Gambert, & Duthie (1981)	N = 20 residents in 190-bed skilled nursing facility	Descriptive study (6 months) on placement of patients	Placement of the mentally incompetent resident with one who is competent may result in alteration of competent patient's emotional status
Zimmer, Watson, & Treat (1984)	N = 1139, random sample (33%) of 42 patients in a skilled nursing facility	Descriptive epidemiological model	Analysis yielded 64.2% with significant behavior problems; 66.5% had diagnosis of organic brain syndrome
Williams, Campbell, Raynor, Mlynarczyk, & Ward (1985)	N = 57 hospitalized elderly with hip fractures	Quasi-experimental 2-group design; treatment was preventive program designed by nursing	Treatment group resulted in lower acute postoperative confusion—51.5% in control group & 43% in treatment group; effective interventions included continuity of care, correcting sensory deficits, & clarification
Roberts & Lincoln (1988)	N = 172, random sample of 94 hospitalized & 78 institutionalized patients, ages 65-99	Theory testing; path analysis to test magnitude of relationship between variables related to confusion	Environmental deficits contributed to cognitive disturbance in institutionalized groups; neural function associated with dysfunction in both groups
Foreman (1989)	N = 71 patients over age 60 admitted to medical intensive care units	Pre-test & posttest quasi-experimental design to test mental status	38% of the patients developed confusion within 6 days of admission; patients who were confused had more medications, more abnormal lab values, & less interaction with significant others

Other selected references in this area: (Bernier & Small, 1988; Burgio, Jones, Butler, & Engle, 1988; Campbell, Williams, & Mlynarczyk, 1986; Chisolm, Denniston, Igrisan, & Barbus, 1982; Clendaniel & Fleishell, 1989; Doyle, Dunn, Thadian, & Lenihan, 1986; Eaton, Mitchell-Bonair, & Friedmann, 1986; Eisenberg & Tierney, 1985; Evans, 1987; Foreman, 1987; Hussian & Brown, 1987; Johnson & Gueldner, 1989; Jones, 1985; Langland & Panicucci, 1983; Lincoln, 1984; Maas & Buckwalter, 1988; Maddox, 1990; Mayers & Griffin, 1990; McCrackin & Fitzwater, 1989; Negley, 1986; Negley & Manley, 1990; Niemoller, 1990; Palmateer & McCartney, 1985; Richter, 1989; Rosswurm, 1989; Ryden & Knopman, 1989; Shomaker, 1987; Struble & Sivertsen, 1987; Vermeersch, 1987; Williams, Campbell, Raynor, Muscholt, Mlynarczyk, & Crane, 1985; Williams, Holloway, Winn, Wolanin, Lawler, Westwick, & Chinn, 1979; Williams, Ward, & Campbell, 1988; Winger & Schirm, 1989; Young, Muir-Nash, & Ninos, 1988)

Table 4.14
TECHNICAL QUALITY OF CARE: BEREAVEMENT (Selected References)

Reference	Study Population	Design	Findings
Gass (1987a)	N = 100 widows in community, mean age 71	Descriptive correlational design to describe successful & unsuccessful coping	Successful coping strategies included participation in social groups, learning new skills, review of spouse's death, & sensing of deceased's presence; unsuccessful strategies included taking antidepressants, sedatives, & tranquilizers
Remondet & Hansson (1987)	N = 75 widowed, unremarried women ages 60-90	Descriptive correlational using 4 measures	Grief resolution index provided reliable way to identify individuals experiencing bereavement-related stress; screening used to pick up early signs & symptoms; data used for prevention
Warner (1987)	N = 30 widows mean age 66 & 30 widowers mean age 64; rural community	Descriptive correlational design using qualitative interviews & 2 surveys	Significant relationship between grief profiles & social support; loss of control & somatization covaried with social support
Farnsworth (1988)	N = 219: 109 divorced & 110 widowed, over age 50, random select	Cross-sectional design to investigate influence of self-esteem on well-being	Individual's perception of health was the major indicator of well-being, regardless of widowhood or divorce; divorced had more confusion, guilt, & anger; widowed experienced more depression; self-esteem influenced well-being

Other selected references in this area: (Constantino, 1988; Gass, 1988; Gass & Chang, 1989; Gass, 1987b; Herth, 1990; Kirschling & Austin, 1988; Richter, 1987; Valanis & Yeaworth, 1982; Valanis, Yeaworth, & Mullis, 1987)

Table 4.15
TECHNICAL QUALITY OF CARE: RELOCATION (Selected References)

Reference	Study Population	Design	Findings
Petrou & Obenchain (1987)	N = 101 patients: 50% in treatment group for relocation & 50% usual care	Experimental design, 2-group posttest	Treatment group had fewer incidents of negative health indicators, including fever, pneumonia, upper respiratory infection, urinary tract infection, & admission to hospital; occurred regardless of age
McCracken (1987)	N = 75 women ages 65-70 who relocated to age-segregated retirement villages	Descriptive study to analyze outcomes of relocation	A decrease in possessions that accompanies relocation increases difficulty of relocation; loss of continuity with life, sense of self, & self-identity also occurs
Rantz & Egan (1987)	N = 91 residents relocated in nursing home	Quasi-experimental design using step-wise regression analysis & evaluation of subsequent program implementation	Anger & anxiety before relocation increased the risk of death for people with deteriorating conditions & depression
Brooke (1988)	N = 44 adults newly admitted to intermediate care facility	Longitudinal participant-observer design; assessed variables such as falls, mental state, family interaction, & medication	Whether relocation was voluntary influenced outcomes; if voluntary, more positive outcomes; 3 phases were identified; residents returned to disorganization with crisis

Other selected references in this area: (Amenta, Weiner, & Amenta, 1984; Bellin, 1990; Brooke, 1989; Chenitz, 1983; Engle, 1985; King, Dimond, & McCance, 1987)

Table 4.16
ISSUES SURROUNDING QUALITY OF DEATH: END-OF-LIFE DIRECTIVES (Selected References)

Reference	Study Population	Design	Findings
Bedell & Delbanco (1984)	N = 157 physicians & 154 patients and/or family members	Retrospective design to study the extent to which patients or family were involved with decision making related to cardiopulmonary resuscitation	Only 10% of patients & 21% of family members had discussed end-of-life directives with their MD or house staff, even though 68% of MDs had formed an opinion about the wishes of the patient; beliefs of patients who survived & physicians had only weak agreement correlation relating to CPR wishes
Lewandowski, Daly, McClish, Juknialis, & Younger (1985)	N = 68 patients with do-not-resuscitate (DNR) orders	Descriptive design to assess changes in aggressiveness of care & resource consumption after DNR order	93% of patients with DNR orders remained on vents, although none were started after DNR order; resource consumption dropped, but physical dependency needs remained intense
Bedell, Pelle, Mahr, & Cleary (1986)	N = 521 patients with DNR orders	Descriptive exploratory design to examine compliance with policy & patient input into DNR decision	Only 22% of patients were involved in the decision to have DNR order
Justin & Johnson (1989)	N = 100 patients admitted for elective surgery	Descriptive survey design to examine patient's wishes related to end-of-life directives & response to survey on topic	Most patients reacted positively to survey; 82% wanted the survey placed on health chart; some asked to forward copy to MD; 15% identified anxiety associated with completing survey

Other selected references in this area: (Cassells, 1988; Jezierski, 1988; Shelley, Zahorchak, & Gambrill, 1987)

Table 4.17			
TECHNICAL QUALITY OF CARE: FAMILY CAREGIVER ISSUES (Selected References)			
Reference	**Study Population**	**Design**	**Findings**
Corbin & Strauss (1984)	N = 60 couples with 1 spouse with chronic illness	Grounded theory	When coordination & collaboration are present, outcome is harmony; suggestions for nursing treatment include better communication, identifying source of conflict, & heightening open awareness
Phillips & Rempusheski (1985)	N = 29 community health care providers who devoted 50% of their time to care for frail elderly & families	Theory-building to formulate model to identify decision-making model	4-stage model was developed which provides basis for how to intervene with elder abuse & neglect
Baillie, Norbeck, & Barnes (1988)	N = 87 family caregivers providing care at home for family without pay	Descriptive study	Elder's condition, length of caregiving, & perceived level of social suppoort explained 50% of variance in psychological distress & depression; caregivers at highest risk for depression are those caring for mentally impaired elderly for extended length of time
Robinson (1989)	N = 78 wives serving as primary caregivers, plus 75 significant others	Descriptive structured interviews	Caregiver health & attitude toward seeking help were significant predictors of depression; past marital adjustment predictor of subjective burden

Other selected references in this area: (Bowers, 1987; Bryant, Candland, & Lowenstein, 1974; Cora, 1986; Ethridge & Lamb, 1989; Fulmer & Ashley, 1989; Gaynor, 1989; Given, King, Collins, & Given, 1988; Given, Stommel, Collins, King, & Given, 1990; Graham, 1989; Johnson & Maguire, 1989; Kalayjian, 1989; Lund, Feinhauer, & Miller, 1985; Phillips & Rempusheski, 1986; Robinson, 1989; Robinson, 1988; Sexton, 1984; Sexton & Munro, 1985; Shomaker, 1987; Wilson, 1989a; Wilson, 1989b)

Table 4.18
TECHNICAL QUALITY OF CARE: NURSING HOME PLACEMENT DECISION CRITERIA
(Selected References)

Reference	Study Population	Design	Findings
Smallegan (1981)	N = 34 patients admitted to nursing home	Qualitative descriptive interviews	Fewer than 50% of patients were decision-makers in their own nursing home placement; ambulation difficulty most common problem; hospitalization was precursor in ⅔ of cases
Smallegan (1985)	N = 288 persons admitted to nursing home	Retrospective design to describe population being admitted	For those being admitted to nursing home, men were caregivers almost ⅔ as often as women; major problems precipitating admission were confusion & ambulation difficulty
Goto & Braun (1987)	N = patients involved in Hawaii's Nursing Home Without Walls (NHWW) program	Retrospective comparative analysis of cost & patient outcomes	Cost per patient day of NHWW care was 61% of average cost of institutionalized nursing home patients; NHWW patients improved in more ADL & mobility items than nursing home patients
Kaplan (1988)	N = 42 patients with dementia	Observation & survey to assess variables associated with placement	Best predictor of nursing home placement was family stress level

Other selected references in this area: (Humphreys, Mason, Guthrie, Liem, & Stern, 1988; Jamieson, 1990; Jamieson, Campbell, & Clarke, 1989; Johnson & Werner, 1982; Matthiesen, 1989; McCann, 1988; Mumma, 1987; Schultz & Magilve, 1988; Schultz & McGlone, 1977; Sullivan & Armignacco, 1979; Worcester & Quayhagen, 1983)

Table 4.19
TECHNICAL QUALITY OF CARE: NURSING STAFF ISSUES (Selected References)

Reference	Study Population	Design	Findings
Ebersole (1985b)	N = 46 nurse administrators	Descriptive study on identification of gerontological nurse practitioners' outcomes	Increased cost containment & quality improvement with use of nurse practitioners
Campbel (1985)	Long-term care facility	Descriptive study of primary nursing	75% reduction in incidence of decubiti; nurse turnover rate decreased by 29%; decrease in death rate by 18%; increase in patient discharges by 11%
Chandler, Rachal, & Kazelskis (1986)	N = 101 random sample of nursing staff at 2 long-term care facilities	Descriptive study examining attitudes toward elderly according to position	Skilled nursing employees are not as negative toward elderly as literature might suggest; RNs most positive; LPNs most negative
Loveridge & Heineken (1988)	N = 400 nursing staff	Descriptive correlational pretest & posttest examining the number of times nurses communicated with residents of a long-term care facility following in-service training	Significant relationship between nurse job satisfaction & quality of care; communication response with residents by nurses occurred in 83% of interactions; increased to 89% after in-service training

Other selected references in this area: (Allen, 1989; Caudill & Patrick, 1989; Chaisson, Beutler, Yost, & Allender, 1984; Chisholm, Deniston, Igrisan, & Barbus, 1982; Cronin & Harrison, 1988; Cuyu & Caltreider, 1987; Doering, 1983; Ebersole, 1985a; Glasspoole & Aman, 1990; Gomez, Otto, Blattstein, & Gomez, 1985; Haff, McGowan, Potts, & Streekstra, 1988; Harris, 1988; Heater, Becker, & Olson, 1988; Huss, Buckwalter, & Stolley, 1988; Johnson, 1987; Jones, 1985; Knaus, Draper, Wagner, & Zimmerman, 1986; Kovner, 1986; Langland & Panicucci, 1983; Lincoln, 1984; Linn, Gurel, & Linn, 1977; Mech, 1980; Miller & Russel, 1980; Palmer, McCormick, & Langford, 1989; Rosendahl & Ross, 1982; Schultz & Magilve, 1988; Schultz & McGlone, 1977; Shelly, Zahorchak, & Gambrill, 1987; Steffes & Thralow, 1985; Woolferk, 1989; Yauger, 1984)

5

Intervention programs to improve the quality of geriatric care

Moving elderly patients and their families from dependence to independence as efficiently and effectively as possible is a challenge to the nation's health care system. Professional nurses meet this challenge by practicing according to the basic tenet of Virginia Henderson—to assist individuals and families in the performance of those activities contributing to health or its recovery (or to a peaceful death) that they would perform unaided if they had the necessary strength, will, or knowledge; and to help individuals and families to be independent of such assistance as soon as possible (American Nurses Association, 1980).

How can individuals or their families be helped to help themselves? What is the professional nurse to provide in the process? Whether a patient and family need this nursing assistance in the hospital, nursing home, or home care setting, valid and reliable nursing research data are sought to answer these questions.

The Rubenstein, Rubenstein, and Josephson paper used its section on intervention programs to describe special programs that improve the processes and outcomes of care for elderly persons—such as geriatric assessment, home visit, innovative nursing home residential care, home care, respite care, and case management programs. Many of these programs identified nurses and other health professionals as participants. However, there was minimal description of nonphysician activities. The authors agree with the Rubenstein, Rubenstein, and Josephson paper's finding that further research needs to be conducted in this area, and suggest that nurses and nursing care be major research variables in each study.

In this section, two specific general project areas are identified and described, followed by descriptions of selected quality assurance and effectiveness programs. Two significant studies of major program interventions include a) the U.S. Office of Technology Assessment's (OTA) study on nurse practitioners, physicians' assistants, and certified nurse midwives; and b) The Robert Wood Johnson Foundation Teaching Nursing Home Program.

The major conclusion of the OTA study was:

> Given that the quality of care provided by nurse practitioners and physician assistants within their areas of competence is equivalent to the quality of comparable services provided by physicians, using nurse practitioners and physician assistants rather than physicians to provide certain services would appear to be cost-effective from a societal perspective.

The studies reviewed in the OTA report concluded that most primary care traditionally provided by physicians can be delivered by nurse practitioners and physician assistants. The OTA study noted that physician assistants tend to function primarily as substitutes for physicians, generally providing only services that physicians provide. However, nurse practitioners are likely to provide protocol-directed services usually provided by physicians, as well as services generally provided by nurses.

The Robert Wood Johnson Foundation Teaching Nursing Home Program has been described as an experiment in social change. The project sought to radically alter professional attitudes about care of the frail elderly. The teaching nursing home was designed from the point of view of the university school of nursing. At this time, there are only preliminary evaluation data.

In the Rutgers Teaching Nursing Home, a system to monitor clinical outcomes was put into place early in the project. After one year of project implementation with a professional staff, there was a 50% decrease in decubitus ulcers, a 23% decrease in use of physical restraints, a 2% decrease in the infection rate with no multiple site infections, a 24% decrease in the use of enemas, a 13% decrease in the number of residents who were totally dependent on a caregiver for their hygiene needs, and 18% fewer transfers to acute care facilities. Over time, bowel and bladder control increased and the use of laxatives and psychotropic drugs decreased.

A change in administration and a decision to substitute nonprofessional personnel for licensed personnel, however, caused Rutgers to move its teaching nursing home. The consequences were significant. The number of persons who fed themselves independently dropped from 27% to 6%; the use of physical restraints increased from 59% to 75%; and bowel incontinence increased from 54% to 74%. Bowel training dropped from 63% to 16%, and regular enema and cathartic use increased from 28% to 45%. Not surprisingly, the clinical indicators that maintained their quality gains were those accorded priority by Medicaid surveyors and routinely monitored by the government, such as decubiti, use of catheters, and incidence of infections.

The rationale behind the Robert Wood Johnson Foundation Teaching Nursing Home Program was that additional costs incurred by strengthening professional nursing in nursing homes could be offset by savings achieved through reducing the use of hospital care and shortening the length of nursing home stays for some patients. Evaluation underway includes a study of patient outcomes, case mix, costs of care, and comparisons between teaching nursing homes and traditional nursing homes. Part of the program also offered increased opportunities for the conduct of clinical research on decubitus ulcers, urinary incontinence, and prevention of falls among the elderly.

Quality Assurance Programs

Health professionals are seriously questioning how to assess and assure quality in a comprehensive yet efficient way. The range of programs in use illustrates the variability and adaptability of quality assurance methods. If quality indicators are assessed and deficiencies in care are identified without actions to correct those deficiencies, there is little chance that improvement will occur. The *assurance* component of quality assurance occurs when corrective action is taken and reassessment indicates improvement (see Table 5.1). For example, the management of principal conditions, hazardous mobility, behavior and constipation ceased to be problems in one study of 60 nursing homes that were assigned nursing quality assurance actions following an audit.

Nine studies described nursing research on the development and testing of comprehensive quality measurement tools (see Table 5.2). Investigators have experimented with using a variety of indicators, including compliance with ethical policies, pain control in hospice programs, preoperative teaching, accuracy of height and weight measurement, use of Bucks traction, and urinary incontinence documentation.

One study described the development of scaled patient outcome criteria for assessment in an extended care facility. The American Nurses Association's *Standards of Nursing Practice* (1973) and *Standards and Scope of Gerontological Nursing Practice* (1987) provide most useful categories—ingestion of food, fluid and nutrient intake, elimination of body wastes, excesses in fluid, locomotion, exercise, regulatory mechanisms, etc.

The testing of the validity and reliability of comprehensive quality assurance tools is a research concern to nurses. Two fairly reliable tools have been developed for assessing case-managed long-term care.

A correlational study of two widely used nursing quality assessment tools (QualPacs and Methodology for Monitoring Quality of Nursing Care, or Rush-Medicus) indicated that each measures a different dimension, indicating that nursing care is complex and multidimensional. Nurses are testing the applicability of a modified Rush-Medicus tool in nursing home settings. Investigators are testing a scaled general symptom distress scale in five home care programs. A hospital Adverse Patient Occurrence Inventory (APOI) tool is proving to be a reliable indicator of hospital costs and length of stay. In Wisconsin, systems engineers and nurses pilot-tested components of a nursing home quality assurance tool for interrater reliability and found positive correlations with general assessments. Two additional studies support the value of monitoring incident reports and providing audit feedback to staff.

Programs Which Improve the Effectiveness of Health Care

This section presents an overview of effectiveness studies (see Table 5.3), most of which are directed to identify patients' self-care deficits and nursing practice effectiveness in self-care performance.

Four studies identified patients' general discharge needs following hospitalization, and nursing effectiveness in fulfilling those needs. In one descriptive pilot study, nurses had patients administer their own medications in the hospital under supervision prior to discharge. The study delineated techniques for conducting such a program safely and effectively. A second study used a discharge questionnaire to identify areas of inadequate teaching. A rehabilitation program was developed, and discharge questionnaires confirmed all deficiencies were remedied.

Two of the studies evaluated patients' perceptions of their discharge needs. Patients identified discharge needs in 15 areas. 27% had received referrals for home services. Patients identified that their needs had been met by the discharge planning process 93% of the time.

Two studies evaluated patient compliance following a structured cardiac rehabilitation program. Compliance was not related to spouse support, demography, or illness variables, but was significantly related to remaining in an ongoing rehabilitation program.

Pulmonary rehabilitation effectiveness has been documented in three experimental design studies. Following a structured instructional program for patients with chronic obstructive pulmonary disease, compliance with their regimen significantly increased, respiratory muscle strength increased, exercise tolerance increased, and symptoms decreased. Similarly, four studies of structured teaching for patients with hypertension resulted in life-style modifications; blood pressure reduction; reduced anxiety; and an improvement in beliefs in personal control of health, knowledge of medications, and self-care behavior. Various other nursing modalities have been tested, including relaxation therapy for control of hypertension and prior to anxiety-producing procedures, testing and programming related to ear care and hearing, crisis intervention counseling, and health assessments at health fairs.

Questions arise as to whether a program is financially justifiable and concerning the kinds of health care for which people are willing to pay. Health professionals have difficulty quantifying the cost-effectiveness of health promotion activities, especially for the elderly—whose overriding concern may be functionality, quality of life, and self-control, rather than longevity. One program to provide health maintenance care to 1,200 elderly living in three rural communities began on a budget of $500 in 1972. By 1978, the budget had grown to $40,000—appropriated by local government and the United Way.

Fall Prevention Programs

The consequences of falls for many elderly can be fractures, immobility, or death. Aged patients with fractures show poor health, unrecognized visual disorders, and pyramidal tract disorders. Falls can occur from stroke, loss of balance, disability, motor abnormalities, and errors in judgment. Poorly adjusted, confused, or agitated individuals are at highest risk.

Restrictions on elderly persons in order to reduce falls, however, can result in loss of independence, decreased quality of life, and increased physical mobility problems. In one study, 67% of the patients who fell had been restrained. Reduction in the use of restraints and increased use of other preventive measures resulted in a decrease in falls. Nursing research on falls has focused on identification of patients at risk for falling and practices that can reduce the incidence of falls without compromising self-sufficiency.

Examples of Fall Prevention Programs

Seven studies on falls, conducted in hospitals, were reviewed. All but one demonstrated a significant reduction in patient falls following a fall prevention program (see Table 5.4). A similar nursing home study described a 21% reduction in falls following monthly reporting and tracking of incidents. One report on a special nursing project identified an 81.75% reduction in falls on a geropsychiatric unit over a two-year period.

Risk Factors for Elderly Who Fall

Eight studies documented that the hospitalized patients most likely to fall are over 75 years of age; in generally poor health; or have diagnosed neurologic deficits, impaired mobility, or confusion (see Table 5.5). Most falls occur in patients' rooms. Depression and substance abuse also are precipitating factors. There is conflicting evidence regarding the effects of medications on incidence of falls. Fall prevention programs include risk assessment; environmental alterations; and patient, family, and staff education.

Intervention Programs to Improve the Mental Status of the Cognitively Impaired Elderly

Over 20 studies used control group comparisons to investigate cognitively impaired elderly persons (see Tables 5.6 to 5.9). The therapy objectives included reduction of confusion, reality orientation, and remotivation. The testing instruments most frequently used were the Mini-Mental Status Test and the Modified Crighton Geriatric Rating Scale (MCGRE) behavioral function improvement tools. Reality orientation programs were found to improve socialization, self-care, and quality of life (see Table 5.6). Three studies reported nonsignificant results. Moderately confused patients tended to respond more favorably than severely confused patients to reality-orientation programs.

Seven studies addressed reminiscence programs. On the whole, results were quite positive (see Table 5.7). Significant improvements in cognitive functioning, socialization, self-esteem, and morale were documented. Depressed patients did appear to have significant improvement. The therapy was useful as a means of interaction with mentally impaired elderly clients.

Four studies on the value of music and movement therapy all cited positive outcomes (see Table 5.8). One four-month program reported improved ability to relate to others, even among the regressed client group. Movement therapy was not effective with agitated clients.

The beneficial role of pets for both well elderly and cognitively impaired elderly is receiving increasing attention (see Table 5.9). At present, this research remains exploratory. In one study, the petting of a companion dog decreased systolic and diastolic blood pressure. Another study found that pets may alleviate loneliness, depression, feelings of helplessness, and social withdrawal. Two other studies, however, found no relationship between pet ownership and psychological well-being or health. Although a pet can be beneficial, this positive effect is absent at the time of another severe loss for elderly persons. More research is suggested before conclusions can be drawn satisfactorily.

Reality orientation, reminiscence, and music and pet therapy, on the whole, have demonstrated positive effects on the cognitive statuses of selected mentally impaired elderly populations. The mixed research results from noninstitutional settings may indicate that dependent nursing home clients are more sensory deprived than are active, involved elderly, who may perceive these activities as inappropriate. □

Table 5.1
**INTERVENTION PROGRAMS TO IMPROVE THE QUALITY OF GERIATRIC CARE: QUALITY
ASSURANCE PROGRAMS (Selected References)**

Reference	Study Population	Design	Findings
Hart & Sliefert (1983)	Long-term care facility	Descriptive study identifying outcomes of quality assurance program	Decrease in number of incidents in every category except falls during 12-month study period of long-term care facility; incidents reduced by 21%
Petrucci, McCormick, & Scheve (1987)	N = 197 patient records	Retrospective descriptive study identifying different quality assurance documentation systems	Results showed variation in documented data depending on form used; authors suggest computerization for consistency
Mohide, Tugwell, Caulfield, Chambers, Dunnett, Baptiste, Byne, Patterson, Rudnick, & Pill (1988)	N = 60 nursing homes randomly assigned to receive new quality assurance intervention	Experimental design	Improved management of principal conditions, hazardous mobility, & constipation using quality assurance interventions
Whiteneck (1988)	Inpatient setting	Descriptive study; quality assurance implementation integrating ethics	Program monitors end-of-life directives as part of quality assurance to enhance data base & assess needs

Other selected references in this area: (Bohnet, 1982; Distel, 1982; Gustafson, Fiss, Fraybach, Smelser, & Hiles, 1980; McMillan & Jasmund, 1985; Mezey, Lynaugh, & Cherry, 1984; Neubauer, LeSage, & Roberts, 1989)

Table 5.2
INTERVENTION PROGRAMS TO IMPROVE THE QUALITY OF GERIATRIC CARE: EXAMPLES OF QUALITY ASSURANCE TOOLS (Selected References)

Reference	Study Population	Design	Findings
Ventura, Hageman, Slakter, & Fox (1982)	N = 273 hospitalized patients	Correlational design to examine QualPacs & Rush-Medicus	Results indicate that instruments measure different dimensions underscoring that quality of nursing care is complex & multidimensional
Panniers & Newlander (1986)	N = 462 patient charts	Instrument testing of Adverse Patient Occurrences Inventory (APOI)	Significant positive correlation between APOI, hospital costs, & length of stay
Lalonde (1987)	N = 150 patients in 5 home care agencies	Instrument development & testing	Instrument development of the General Symptom Distress scale; high incidence of symptom distress; good screening device for further investigation of agency
Howe, Coulton, Almon, & Sandrick (1980a)	Inpatient setting	Instrument development, with American Nurses Association's *Standards of Nursing Practice* used as framework	Outcome criteria include ingestion of food, elimination, locomotion, exercise, regulatory mechanisms, interpersonal relating, & self-actualization

Other selected references in this area: (Abrahams & Lamb, 1988; Hewitt, LeSage, Roberts, & Ellor, 1985; Howe, Coulton, & Almon, 1980b; Panniers & Tomkiewicz, 1985; Thee & Obrecht, 1984)

Table 5.3
INTERVENTION PROGRAMS TO IMPROVE THE EFFECTIVENESS OF HEALTH CARE
(Selected References)

Reference	Study Population	Design	Findings
Perry (1981)	N = 20 patients with chronic obstructive pulmonary disease	Descriptive study to test and examine effects of pulmonary rehabilitation program	Significant decrease in number of symptoms, including shortness of breath, wheezing, tightness in chest, & difficulty expectorating phlegm; number of therapies used also increased significantly
Jordan-Marsh & Neutra (1985)	N = 337 community participants, 66% between ages 50-70	Quasi-experimental pre-test & posttest design to test effectiveness of a life-style modification program on cardiovascular parameters	Significant changes in locus of control scores from admission to discharge; significant inverse relationships between powerful other scores & changes in triglycerides & cholesterol/high density lipids
Larson (1986)	N = 22 patients with moderate to severe chronic obstructive pulmonary disease; randomly assigned to 2 treatment groups	Experimental 2-group pre-test & posttest design; groups exercised inspiratory muscles with threshold resistance—one at 15% & one at 30% individual maximum load	Group using 30% improved significantly in inspiratory muscle strength, respiratory muscle endurance, & general exercise tolerance; 15% improved only in maximal inspiratory pressure (both significant)
Goodman (1989)	N = 63 patients with chronic obstructive pulmonary disease, 33 in control & 30 in treatment group	Experimental 2-group design using implementation of pulmonary rehabilitation program for treatment group	The treatment group demonstrated significantly higher compliance with regimen, as well as higher psychosocial adjustment

Other selected references in this area: (Dinsmore, 1979; Furukawa, 1981; Harper, 1984; Hilbert, 1985; Kobza, 1983; Krommings & Ostwald, 1987: Macauley, Murray, & Ellis, 1980; McPhee, Frank, Lewis, Bush, & Smith, 1983; Naylor, 1990; Pender, 1985; Scura, 1988; Small & Walsh, 1988; Stanley, 1988; Sullivan & Armignacco, 1979; Uman & Hazard, 1981; Wilson, Patterson, & Alford, 1989)

Table 5.4
INTERVENTION PROGRAMS TO IMPROVE THE QUALITY OF GERIATRIC CARE: EXAMPLES OF FALL PREVENTION PROGRAMS (Selected References)

Reference	Study Population	Design	Findings
Innes & Turman (1983)	N = all falls in an acute care setting before and after intervention	Quasi-experimental pre-test and posttest design to identify outcomes of a nursing intervention program	Falls decreased by 50% after workshop & development of screening tool to identify high-risk patients
Campbell, Williams, & Mlynarczyk (1986)	N = 170 hospitalized patients on orthopedic units	Quasi-experimental design testing outcome of confusion on 4 units where nursing program was implemented	Incidence of confusion related to falls decreased 44-55% on 3 of 4 units
Hernandez & Miller (1986)	N = all fall incidents on gero-psychiatric unit & comparison of falls postintervention	Quasi-experimental pre-test & posttest design	Fall rate decreased 42.3% the first year & 39.4% the second year following intervention program implementation
Hendrich (1988)	N = all patients who fell in an acute care hospital and matched control group	2-group quasi-experimental pre-test and posttest design	Implementation of fall prevention program reduced falls by 50-75%

Other selected references in this area: (Innes, 1985; Rainville, 1984; Spellbring, Gannon, Klechner, & Conway, 1988)

Table 5.5
INTERVENTION PROGRAMS TO IMPROVE THE QUALITY OF GERIATRIC CARE: RISK FACTORS FOR ELDERLY WHO FALL (Selected References)

Reference	Study Population	Design	Findings
Hart & Sliefert (1983)	N = falls occurring in 12-month period in 1 long-term care facility	Descriptive identification of risk factors	High-risk factors included age over 80, diagnosis of senility, impaired mobility, & confusion; patient rooms were most frequent location of fall
Janken, Reynolds, & Swiech (1986)	N = 331 patients over age 60 who fell during hospitalization, compared with 300 randomly drawn patients who did not fall	2-group descriptive design for comparative analysis	Fall patients can be identified if risk factors are identified & screened for upon hospital admission; risk factors include general weakness & decreased mobility
Johnston (1988)	N = 46 residents ages 65-98 residing in independent living facilities	Descriptive exploratory design using interviews & observations	Almost half of residents had experienced 1 or more falls in previous year; residents were classified into 2 qualitative categories: "slow watchers" who watched, waited, & proceeded slowly were nonfallers; "planners" who changed their environment & avoided danger were most likely to fall
Llewellyn, Martin, Shekleton, & Firlit (1988)	N = 429; 120 pre-test & 309 posttest, mean ages 64.8 & 69.4	Quasi-experimental pre-test & posttest design; identification of risk factors	Incidence of falls increased in second test; influencing risk factors were found to be increased patient acuity & decreased nurse staffing

Other selected references in this area: (Berryman, Gaskin, Jones, Tolley, & MacMullen, 1989; Johnston, 1987; Morse, Dixon, & Tylko, 1985; Walshe & Rosen, 1979)

Table 5.6
INTERVENTION PROGRAMS TO IMPROVE THE MENTAL STATUS OF THE COGNITIVELY IMPAIRED ELDERLY: REALITY ORIENTATION, REMOTIVATION, AND RESOCIALIZATION (Selected References)

Reference	Study Population	Design	Findings
Voelkel (1978)	N = 20 elderly nursing home residents randomly assigned to reality orientation or resocialization groups	Experimental 2-group design	Groups showed significant improvement on the SPMSQ scale, with resocialization group showing greater improvement; no changes found on Lawton Physical Self Maintenance Scale
Hogstel (1979)	N = 40 randomly selected confused elderly who were randomly assigned to a reality orientation control group	Experimental pre-test & posttest design	Results nonsignificant, although moderately confused patients improved more than slightly or severely confused patients
Nodhturft & Sweeney (1982)	N = 41 randomly selected nursing home residents who were randomly assigned to treatment or control groups	Experimental 2-group design	Treatment group which focused on reality orientation & reminiscence showed significant improvement on the Mental Status Schedule
Janssen & Giberson (1988)	N = 14 participants in adult day care	Quasi-experimental design testing effect of remotivation sessions	Socialization improved; sensory stimulation for cognitvely impaired elderly increased; group identification & cohesiveness increased

Other selected references in this area: (Citrin & Dixon, 1977; Cornbleth & Cornbleth, 1979; Gray & Stevenson, 1980; Hanley, 1981; Mulcahy & Rosa, 1981; Nagley, 1986; Reeve & Ivison, 1985; Robb, Stegman, & Wolanin, 1986; Seaman & Roth, 1989; Settles, 1985; Tolbert, 1984; Zepelin, Wolfe, & Kleinplatz, 1981)

Table 5.7
INTERVENTION PROGRAMS TO IMPROVE THE MENTAL STATUS OF THE COGNITIVELY IMPAIRED ELDERLY: REMINISCENCE (Selected References)

Reference	Study Population	Design	Findings
Hughston & Merriam (1982)	N = 105 residents living in housing for the elderly	Experimental pre-test & posttest design	Reminiscence group had significantly improved scores of cognitive functioning
Baker (1985)	N = 8 mentally impaired elderly adults at day care center	Quasi-experimental design to test reminiscence therapy	Evaluation reported evidence of improvement in verbal interaction, eye contact, touch, smiles, accepting leadership, & participation; sense of group cohesiveness & empathy
Schafer (1985)	N = 30 nursing homes randomly assigned to treatment & control groups; 185 patients from stratified random sample	Experimental pre-test & posttest design	Results indicate that reminiscence groups are beneficial to the extent that patients are able to exert control over the nature of the program
Lappe (1987)	N = 83 patients in long-term care facilities, mean age 82.6, randomly assigned	Experimental posttest design only	Group sessions utilizing reminiscence increase self-esteem scores to a greater degree than group sessions using current events

Other selected references in this area: (Parsons, 1984; Perrotta & Meacham, 1981-82; Walker, 1984)

Table 5.8
INTERVENTION PROGRAMS TO IMPROVE THE MENTAL STATUS OF THE COGNITIVELY IMPAIRED ELDERLY: MUSIC AND MOVEMENT THERAPY (Selected References)

Reference	Study Population	Design	Findings
Kartman (1977)	N = 13, 8 patients physically regressed & 5 patients emotionally regressed	Quasi-experimental design to test intervention	Improvement in residents' ability to relate to each other & enhanced social functioning for both regressed groups
Goldberg & Fitzpatrick (1980)	N = 30 elderly over age 65 living in a nursing home	Experimental 2-group design	Movement therapy sessions conducted over 6 weeks resulted in a significant increase in total morale & attitude toward people their own age; no significant increase in agitation; researchers recommend master's-prepared nurse specialists to perform therapy
Olson (1984)	N = 11 elderly clients in Midwest retirement center	Experimental design to measure responses to music	Marked increments of rhythmic & extremity responses; enhanced state of well-being; enabled retrieval of specific long-term memories
Gueldner & Spradley (1988)	N = 32 elderly living in long-term care facility	Descriptive study to examine effects of outdoor walking	Outdoor walking inexpensive & accessible form of activity that may enable improved state of health

Table 5.9
INTERVENTION PROGRAMS TO IMPROVE THE MENTAL STATUS OF THE COGNITIVELY IMPAIRED ELDERLY: PET THERAPY (Selected References)

Reference	Study Population	Design	Findings
Andrysco (1982)	N = 46 elderly residents, 23 in experimental group & 23 in control group	Experimental design to examine effects of pet in a geriatric facility	A pet in the facility may offer patients a nonthreatening form of tactile contact and nonverbal communication to alleviate loneliness, depression, helplessness, & social withdrawal
Robb & Stegman (1983)	N = 56, 30 aged who did not live with pet & 26 who did live with pet, Veterans Administration home care clients	Exploratory study	No significant differences found related to health variables
Lund, Johnson, Baraki, & Dimond (1984)	N = 104 bereaved widows with pets	Longitudinal descriptive study evaluating influence of pet during bereavement	Beneficial effects that pets have on psychosocial aspects of aging do not appear at time of loss
Baun, Bergstrom, Langston, & Thoma (1984)	N = 24 elderly subjects monitored during 3 measurements	Experimental repeated measures on the same group using 3 different treatments: pet companion dog, pet stranger dog, or reading quietly	Decreased systolic & diastolic blood pressure occurs during petting of companion dog & similar decrease for quiet reading

Other selected references in this area: (Cowles, 1985; Francis & Bahy, 1986; Hamilton, 1985; Kongable, Buckwalter, & Stolley, 1989; Lauton, Moss, & Moles, 1984; Riddick, 1985; Savishinsky, 1985)

6

Important processes of care for elderly persons, as derived from current gerontological nursing textbooks

The Rubenstein, Rubenstein, and Josephson paper included an assessment of important processes of care for elderly persons as derived from current geriatric textbooks. The assessment is contained in Appendix F of that report.

The following similar assessment was made using nursing textbooks.

Important Processes to Be Performed in All Settings

- Assess and promote independence.
- Enable the individual to modify activities of daily living as needed, and as associated with the stages of later life.
- Assess, plan, intervene in, and evaluate care to promote a high level of self-esteem and self-identity.
- Assess, plan, intervene in, and evaluate care to promote effective coping.

- Assess, plan, intervene in, and evaluate care for the following health care needs: rest/activity; sensory experiences; elimination, including incontinence; acute and chronic pain and discomfort; oxygen support; body protection, including temperature and skin condition; mobility; spirituality; and nutrition.
- Promote a safe and secure environment that recognizes the diversity of elderly clients.
- Assess, plan, intervene in, and evaluate care for the mental health needs of the client, including depression, alcoholism, confusion, and dementia.
- Assess signs and symptoms of disease and age-related processes promptly and on an ongoing basis.
- Support the individual through the transitions of later life, including retirement, loss, and grief.
- Modify verbal and nonverbal approaches for varying sensory-perceptual states.
- Provide multidisciplinary and/or interdisciplinary evaluation and rehabilitation services.
- Utilize medications carefully.
- Provide instruction on medication usage and self-administration.
- Assess resources and referrals, including legal resources.
- Assess and promote relationships with significant others.
- Determine caregivers' responsibilities and needs.
- Promote the individual's involvement in decision making regarding health care issues.
- Provide advocacy.

Important Processes to Be Performed in the Hospital

- Promote activity to prevent immobility.
- Prevent and/or minimize risks of hospitalization and iatrogenic conditions and infections, such as pressure sores, confusion, and learned helplessness.
- Diminish the potential for dependency and promote normalcy.

- Include significant others in decision making.
- Allow family or caregivers to participate in the care regime.
- Plan for comprehensive posthospital care.
- Monitor medication effectiveness and reactions.
- Diminish the potential for injury, including frugal usage of physical and chemical restraints.
- Provide education regarding perioperative procedures, conditions, medications, diagnostic procedures, and discharge planning.
- Support the client in life-threatening situations.
- Promote cognitive functioning, including reality orientation, reminiscence, and environmental stimulation or control.
- Monitor vital signs and evaluate changes, particularly hypothermia.
- Monitor fluid and nutrition status.
- Encourage client decision making and honor client wishes regarding care (i.e., living wills).

Important Processes to Be Performed in the Nursing Home

- Provide a social environment to promote a high level of functioning.
- Create a therapeutic environment.
- Prevent potential adverse effects of institutionalization, including dependency, learned helplessness, and decrease in self-esteem.
- Assess, plan, and intervene to deter the potential effects of relocation.
- Assess and provide assistive devices.
- Promote self-care ability utilizing a restorative focus to care delivery.
- Interact frequently with health care team members to modify the plan of care.
- Utilize various approaches to promote cognitive functioning, including reminiscence, life review, reality orientation, and pet therapy.

- Provide comprehensive discharge in transfering to a hospital, other long-term care facility, or the community.

- Allow participation of significant others and facilitate adjustment of family members to placement in the nursing home.

- Provide creative approaches to behavioral management problems associated with chronic conditions, such as wandering, disruptive verbal communication, and agitation.

- Provide education on relevant topics to the elderly.

- Evaluate the effects and consequences of medications.

- Deter immobility.

- Provide for a compassionate and dignified death.

Important Processes to Be Performed in Ambulatory Care and Home Care Programs

- Provide screening programs for high-risk health alterations, including glaucoma, hypertension, hearing, cholesterol, cancer, vision, and alcoholism.

- Provide case management.

- Participate in primary health care management.

- Provide education, particularly in regard to medication usage, care procedures, safety measures, and dietary needs.

- Make home visits to the home-bound elderly.

- Assess the home environment and community resources.

- Assess and provide for the attainment of equipment and assistive devices.

- Provide referrals to support programs, such as adult day care, respite care programs, hospice, and self-help/support groups. □

Bibliography (by Alphabetical Order)

Abrahams, R. and Lamb, S. 1988. Developing reliable assessment in case-managed geriatric long-term care programs. *Quality Review Bulletin* 14(6):179-186.

Adams, M. 1986. Aging: Gerontological nursing research. In *Annual Review of Nursing Research,* vol. 4, eds. H. Werley, J. Fitzpatrick, and R. L. Taunton. New York: Springer.

Adams, F. 1988. Fluid intake: How much do elders drink? *Geriatric Nursing* 9(4):218-221.

Allen, J. 1989. Learning after graduation: Are nurses taking advantage of the resources? *Journal of Gerontological Nursing* 15(8):27-32.

Allman, R.; Walker, J.; Hart, M.; Laprade, C.; Knoll, L.; and Smith, C. 1987. Air fluidized beds or conventional therapy for pressure sores: A randomized trial. *Annals of Internal Medicine* 107:641-648.

Amenta, M.; Weiner, A.; and Amenta, D. 1984. Successful relocation of elderly residents. *Geriatric Nursing:* 5(8):356-360.

American Nurses Association. 1973. *Standards of nursing practice.* Kansas City, Mo.: the Association.

————. 1980. *Nursing: A social policy statement.* Kansas City, Mo.: the Association.

————. 1986. *Standards of home health nursing practice.* Kansas City, Mo.: the Association.

————. 1987. *Standards and scope of gerontological nursing practice.* Kansas City, Mo.: the Association.

————. 1988. *Standards for organized nursing services.* Kansas City, Mo.: the Association.

Andrysco, R. 1982. A study of ethologic and therapeutic factors of pet-facilitated therapy in a retirement nursing community. *Dissertation Abstracts* 43(1):290B.

Athlin, E.; Norberg, A.; Axelsson, K.; Moller, A.; and Nordstrom, G. 1989. Aberrant eating behavior in elderly Parkinsonian patients with and without dementia: Analysis of video-recorded meals. *Research in Nursing and Health* 12(1):12, 41-51.

Bahr, S.R. and Griss, L. 1982. Blood pressure readings and selected parameter relationships in an elderly ambulatory population. *Journal of Gerontological Nursing* 8(3):159-163.

Baigis-Smith, J.; Jakobac-Smith, D.; Rose, M.; and Newman, D. 1989. Managing urinary incontinence in community-residing elderly persons. *The Gerontologist* 29(2):229-233.

Baillie, V.; Norbeck, J.S.; and Barnes, L. 1988. Stress, social support, and psychological distress of family care givers of the elderly. *Nursing Research* 37:217-222.

Baker, N. 1985. Reminiscing in group therapy for self-worth. *Journal of Gerontological Nursing* 11(7):21-24.

Baldini, J. 1981. Knowledge about hypertension in affected elderly persons. *Journal of Gerontological Nursing* 7(9):542-545, 551.

Banasik, J. and Steadman, R. 1987. Effect of position on arterial oxygenation in postoperative coronary revascularization patients. *Heart and Lung* 16(6):652-657.

Barker, J. and Mitteness, L. 1989. Shedding light on nocturia. *Geriatric Nursing* 10(5):239-240.

Bassett, C.; McClamrock, E.; and Schmelzer, M. 1982. A 10-week exercise program for senior citizens. *Geriatric Nursing* 3(2):103-105.

Baun, M.; Bergstrom, N.; Langston, N.; and Thoma, L. 1984. Physiological effects of human/companion animal bonding. *Nursing Research* 33(3):126-129.

Becker, L. and Goodemote, C. 1984. Treating pressure sores with or without antacid. *American Journal of Nursing* 84(3):351-352.

Bedell, S.E. and Delbanco, T.L. 1984. Choices about cardiopulmonary resuscitation in the hospital: When do physicians talk with patients? *New England Journal of Medicine* 310:1089-1093.

Bedell, S.E.; Pelle, D.; Maher, R.L.; and Cleary, P.D. 1986. Do-not-resuscitate orders for critically ill patients in the hospital: How are they used and what is their impact? *Journal of the American Medical Association* 256(2):233-237.

Bellin, C. 1990. Relocating adult day care: Its impact on persons with dementia. *Journal of Gerontological Nursing* 16(3):11-14.

Bergstrom, N.; Braden, B.; Laguzza, A.; and Holman, V. 1987. The Braden scale for predicting pressure sore risk. *Nursing Research* 36(4):205-210.

Bernier, S.L. and Small, N.R. 1988. Disruptive behaviors. *Journal of Gerontological Nursing* 14(2):8-13.

Berryman, E.; Gaskin, D.; Jones, A.; Tolley, F.; and MacMullen G. 1989. Point by point: Predicting elders' falls. *Geriatric Nursing* 10(4):199-201.

Biddle, C. and Biddle, W. 1985. A plastic head cover to reduce surgical heat loss. *Geriatric Nursing* 6(1):39-41.

Black, M.; VanBerkel, C.; Green, E.; Everett, I.; and Krilyk J. 1987. Criteria map—potential for skin breakdown: A quality assurance tool for use in any setting. *Quality Review Bulletin* 15(11):340-345.

Blom, M.F. 1985. Dramatic decrease in decubitus ulcers. *Geriatric Nursing* 6(2):84-87.

Bohnet, N.L. 1982. Quality assessment as an ongoing component of hospice care. *Quality Review Bulletin* 8(5):7-20.

Bowers, B.J. 1987. Intergenerational care giving: Adult caregivers and their aging parents. *Advances in Nursing Science* 9(2):20-31.

Bowsher, J. 1987. Personal control and psychological well-being of institutionalized elders. *Dissertation Abstracts* 48(5):1299B.

Brands, R. 1983. Acceptance of nurses as primary-care providers by retired people. *Advances in Nursing Science* 5(3):37-49.

Braun, J.V. 1987. Failure to thrive aged in nursing home. *Dissertation Abstracts* 48(1):143B.

Bredow, T.S. 1989. Prospective payment policy and the home health care of chronically ill patients. *Dissertation Abstracts* 49(8):3101B.

Brink, C.; Sampselle, C.; Wells, T.; Diokno, A.; and Gillis, G. 1989. A digital test for pelvic muscle strength in older women with urinary incontinence. *Nursing Research* 38(4):196-199.

Bristow, J.; Goldfarb, E.; and Green, M. 1987. Clinitron therapy: Is it effective? *Geriatric Nursing* 8(3):120-124.

Brooke, V. 1988. Adjusting to living in a nursing home: Toward a nursing home intervention model. *Dissertation Abstracts* 48(8): 2259B.

―――. 1989. How elders adjust. *Geriatric Nursing* 10(2):66-68.

Brown, C.S.B. and Stegman, M.R. 1988. Nutritional assessment of surgical patients. *Quality Review Bulletin* 14(10):302-306.

Brown, J.S. and McCreedy, M. 1986. The hale elderly: Health behavior and its correlates. *Research in Nursing and Health* 9(4):317-329.

Brown, M.; Boosinger, J.; Black, J.; and Gaspar, T. 1985. Nursing innovation for prevention of decubitus ulcers in long-term care facilities. *Plastic Surgical Nursing* Summer:57-64.

Brown, M.; Boosinger, J.; Black, J.; Gaspar, T.; and Sather, L. 1982. Nursing innovation for dry skin care of the feet in the elderly: A demonstration project. *Journal of Gerontological Nursing* 8(7):393-395.

Brown, M. and Everett I. 1990. Gentler bowel fitness with fiber. *Geriatric Nursing* 11(1):26-27.

Bryant, N.H.; Candland, L.; and Lowenstein, R. 1974. Comparison of care and cost outcomes for stroke patients with and without home care. *Stroke* 5:54-59.

Buckwalter, K.; Cusack, D.; Stidles, E.; Wadle, K.; and Beaver, M. 1989. Increasing communication ability in aphasic/dysarthric patients. *Western Journal of Nursing Research* 11(6):736-747.

Burckhardt, C.S. 1987. The effect of therapy on the mental health of the elderly. *Research in Nursing and Health* 10(4):277-285.

Burgio, L.; Jones, L.; Butler, F.; and Engel, B. 1988. Behavior problems in an urban nursing home. *Journal of Gerontological Nursing* 14(1):31-34.

Burgio, L.; Jones, L.; and Engel, B. 1988. Studying incontinence in an urban nursing home. *Journal of Gerontological Nursing* 14(4):40-45.

Burnside, I. 1985. *Nursing and the Aged,* 3rd ed. New York: McGraw-Hill.

Butler, F.; Burgio, L.; and Engel, B. 1987. Neuroleptics and behavior: A comparative study. *Journal of Gerontological Nursing* 13(6):15-19.

Byers, P.H. 1985. Effect of exercise on morning stiffness and mobility in patients with rheumatoid arthritis. *Research in Nursing and Health* 8(3):275-281.

Cagawa-Busby, K.; Heltkempr, M.; Hansen, B.; Hanson, R. and Vanderburg, V. 1988. Effects of diet temperature on tolerance of enteral feedings. *Nursing Research* 29(5):276-280.

Cambel, S.D. 1985. Primary nursing: It works in long-term care. *Journal of Gerontological Nursing* 11(12):12-16.

Campbell, E.B.; Williams, M.D.; and Mlynarczyk, S.M. 1986. After the fall: Confusion. *American Journal of Nursing* 86(2):151-154.

Canadian Task Force on the Periodic Health Examination. 1979. *Canadian Medical Association Journal* 121:1193-1254.

Card, D.A. 1987. Underutilization of health care services. *Dissertation Abstracts* 47(8):3292B.

Carnevelli, D. and Patrick, M. 1986. *Nursing management for the elderly.* Philadelphia: J. B. Lippincott.

Cassels, C.; Fortinash, K.; and Eckstein, A. 1981. Retirement: Aspects, responses, andnursing implications. *Journal of Gerontological Nursing* 7(6):355.

Cassels, E.J. 1988. Autonomy in the intensive care unit: The refusal of treatment. *Critical Care Clinics:37.*

Cassels, H.B. 1988. Health beliefs and osteoporosis prevention by menopausal women. *Dissertation Abstracts* 49(6):2123.

Caudill, M. and Patrick, M. 1989. Nursing assistant turnover in nursing homes and need satisfaction. *Journal of Gerontological Nursing* 15(6):24-30.

Chaisson, M.; Beutler, L.; Yost, E.; and Allender, J. 1984. Treating the depressed elderly. *Journal of Psychosocial Nursing* 22(5):25-30.

Chandler, J.; Rachal, J.; and Kazelskis, R. 1986. Attitudes of long-term care nursing personnel toward the elderly. *The Gerontologist* 26(5):551-555.

Chang, B.L. 1978. Generalized expectancy, situational perception, and morale among institutionalized elderly. *Nursing Research* 27(5):316-324.

Chang, B.L.; Uman, G.C.; Linn, L.S.; Ware, J.E.; and Kane, R.L. 1985. Adherence to health care regimens among elderly women. *Nursing Research* 34(1):27-31.

Check, J. and Wurzbach, M. 1984. How elders view learning. *Geriatric Nursing* 5(1):37-39.

Chenitz, W.C. 1983. Entry into a nursing home as a status passage: A theory to guide nursing practice. *Geriatric Nursing* 4(2):92-97.

Chisholm, M.; Lundin, S.; and Wood, J. 1983. Withdrawing digoxin: Worth a try. *Geriatric Nursing* 4(5):290-292.

Chisholm, S.E.; Denniston, O.L.; Igrisan, R.M.; and Barbus, A.J. 1982. Prevalence of confusion in elderly hospitalized patients. *Journal of Gerontological Nursing* 8(2):87-96.

Christian, E.; Dluhy, N.; and O'Neill, R. 1989. Sounds of silence: Coping with hearing loss and loneliness. *Journal of Gerontological Nursing* 15(11):4-9.

Christman, N.J.; McConnell, E.A.; Pfeiffer, C.; Webster, K.K.; Schmitt, M.; and Ries, J.1988. Uncertainty, coping, and distress following myocardial infarction: Transition from hospital to home. *Research in Nursing & Health* 11:71-82.

Chung, S. 1983. Foot care: A health care maintenance program. *Journal of Gerontological Nursing* 9(4):212-227.

Citrin, R.S. and Dixon, D.N. 1977. Reality orientation: A milieu therapy used in an institution for the aged. *The Gerontologist* 17(1):39-43.

Clapin-French, E. 1986. Sleep patterns of aged persons in long-term care facilities. *Journal of Advanced Nursing* 11:57-66.

Clarke, M. 1988. The nursing prevention of pressure sores in hospital and community patients. *Journal of Advanced Nursing* 13:365-373.

Clendaniel, B. and Fleishell, A. 1989. An Alzheimer day care center for nursing home patients. *American Journal of Nursing* 89(7):944-945.

Cleveland, S.A. 1988. Assessment of self-care agency in patients with chronic obstructive pulmonary disease. *Dissertation Abstracts* 49(6):2124B.

Clough, D. and Maurin, J. 1983. ROM versus NRx. *Journal of Gerontological Nursing* 9(5):278-286.

Colanowski, A. and Gunter, L. 1988. Do retired career women exercise? *Geriatric Nursing* 9(6):350-352.

Collard, A.F. 1989. Predicting readmissions of elderly patients to the acute care hospital. *Dissertation Abstracts* 49(8):3101B.

Collard, A.F.; Bachman, S.S.; and Beatrice, D.F. 1985. Acute care delivery for the geriatric patient: An innovative approach. *Quality Review Bulletin* 11(6):180-185.

Colling, J.C. 1985. Elderly nursing home residents' control of activities of daily living and well-being. *Dissertation Abstracts* 46(10):3389-3390B.

Collins, M. 1988. Humor: An informal channel of communication used by institutionalized aged to express feelings of aggression due to personal deficits in power and states. *Dissertation Abstracts* 49(5):1619B.

Collinsworth, R. and Boyle, K. 1989. Nutritional assessment of the elderly. *Journal of Gerontological Nursing* 15(12):17-21.

Committee on Nursing Home Regulation, Institute of Medicine. 1986. *Improving the quality of care in nursing homes.* Washington, D.C.: National Academy Press.

Constantino, R.E. 1988. Comparison of two group interventions for the bereaved. *Image: The Journal of Nursing Scholarship* 20:83-87.

Cora, V.L. 1986. Family life process of intergenerational families with functionally dependent elders. *Dissertation Abstracts* 47(3):568B.

Corbin, J.M. and Strauss, A.L. 1984. Collaboration: Couples working together to manage chronic illness. *Image: The Journal of Nursing Scholarship* 16:109-115.

Cornbleth, T. and Cornbleth, C. 1979. Evaluation of the effectiveness of reality orientation classes in a nursing home unit. *Journal of the American Geriatrics Society* 27(11):522-524.

Cowles, K. 1985. The death of a pet: Human responses to the breaking of the bond. In *Pets and the family,* ed. M. B. Sussman, pp. 135-148. New York: Haworth Press.

Craig, L.L. 1988. Characteristics of older men and their ability to comprehend printed health education materials. *Dissertation Abstracts* 49(4):1088B.

Cronin, S.N. and Harrison, B. 1988. Importance of nurse caring behaviors as perceived by patients after myocardial infarction. *Heart and Lung* 17:374-380.

Cuyu, L. and Caltreider, D.L. 1987. Stressed nurses dealing with incontinent patients. *Journal of Gerontological Nursing* 13(1):27-30.

Daily, E. and Futrell, M. 1989. Retirement attitudes and health status of pre-retired and retired men and women. *Journal of Gerontological Nursing* 15(1):29-32.

Davidson, A.W. and Young, C. 1985. Repatterning of stroke rehabilitation clients following return to life in the community. *Journal of Neurosurgical Nursing* 17:123-128.

Davis, C. and Lentz, M. 1989. Circadian rhythms: Charting oral temperatures to spot abnormalities. *Journal of Gerontological Nursing* 15(4):34-39.

Dean, H. 1988. Multiple instruments for measuring quality of life. In *Instruments for clinical nursing,* ed. M. Frank-Stromborg, pp. 97-105. Norwalk, Conn.: Appleton & Lange.

DeBlase, R.; Badziong, M.R.; and Jones, S.L. 1988. Postintraocular lens implants: Needs of patients. *Geriatric Nursing* 9(6):342-343.

DeMoss, C.J. 1980. Giving intravenous chemotherapy at home. *American Journal of Nursing* 80(12):2188-2189.

Denny, M.; Koren, M.E.; and Wisby, M. 1989. Gynecological health needs of elderly women. *Journal of Gerontological Nursing* 15(1):33-38.

Devey, S. 1990. Older lesbian women: An invisible minority. *Journal of Gerontological Nursing* 16(5):35-39.

Devine, E.C. and Werley, H.H. 1988. Test of the nursing minimum data set: Availability of data and reliability. *Research in Nursing and Health* 11:97-104.

DeVon, H.A. and Powers, M.J. 1984. Health beliefs, adjustment to illness, and control of hypertension. *Research in Nursing and Health* 7(1):10-16.

DeWalt, E. 1975. Effect of timed hygiene measures on oral mucosa in a group of elderly subjects. *Nursing Research* 24:104-108.

Diekmann, J.M. 1984. Use of a dental irrigating device in the treatment of decubitus ulcers. *Nursing Research* 33(5):303-305.

Dietx, M. 1986. Sources of stress among older rural women in North Dakota. *Dissertation Abstracts* 47(4):1486B.

Dinsmore, P. 1979. A health education program for elderly residents in the community. *Nursing Clinics of North America* 14(4):585-593.

Diokno, A.C.; Wells, T.J.; and Brink, C.A. 1987. Urinary incontinence in elderly women: Urodynamic evaluation. *Journal of the American Geriatrics Society* 35:940-946.

Distel, L. 1981. More than chart review. *Quality Review Bulletin* 7(1):26-29.

———. 1982. A nursing quality assurance investigation of orthopedic patient care. *Quality Review Bulletin* 8(10):20-22.

Dixon, J. 1984. Effect of nursing interventions on nutritional and performance status in cancer patients. *Nursing Research* 33:330-335.

Doering, E.R. 1983. Factors influencing inpatient satisfaction with care. *Quality Review Bulletin* 9(10):291-99.

Doering, L. and Dracup, K. 1988. Comparisons of cardiac output in supine and lateral positions. *Nursing Research* 37(2):114-118.

Dolinsky, E. 1987. The relationships of perceived social support and self-disclosure to the morale of older women. *Dissertation Abstracts* 48(3):702B.

Donabedian, A. 1980. *The definition of quality and approaches to its assessment.* Ann Arbor, Mich.: University of Michigan Health Administration Press.

Doyle, G.C.; Dunn, S.I. Thadani, I.; and Lenihan, P. 1986. Investigating tools to aid in restorative care for Alzheimer's patients. *Journal of Gerontological Nursing* 12(9):19-24.

Dressler, D.K.; Smejkal, C.; and Ruffolo, M. L. 1983. A comparison of oral and rectal temperature measurement on patients receiving oxygen by mask. *Nursing Research* 32(6):373-375.

Droessler, D. and Maibusch, R.M. 1982. Development of a nursing care plan for healing and preventing decubiti. *Quality Review Bulletin Special Edition* Spring: 21-25.

Durham, M.L.; Swanson, B.; and Pulford, N. 1986. Effects of tachypnea on oral temperature estimation: A replication. *Nursing Research* 35(4):211-214.

Eaton, M.; Mitchell-Bonair, I.L.; and Friedmann, E. 1986. The effect of touch on nutritional intake of chronic organic brain syndrome patients. *Journal of Gerontology* 41(5):611.

Ebersole, P. 1985a. *Overcoming the bias of ageism in long-term care.* New York: National League for Nursing.

————. 1985b. Gerontological nurse practitioners, past and present. *Geriatric Nursing* 6(4):219-222.

Ebersole, P. and Hess, P. 1981. *Toward healthy aging.* St. Louis: C. V. Mosby.

Edwardson, S.R. 1988. Outcomes of coronary care in the acute care setting. *Research in Nursing and Health* 11(4):215-222.

Eisenberg, M.G. and Tierney, D.O. 1985. Profiling disruptive patient incidents. *Quality Review Bulletin* 11(8):245-248.

Engle, V. 1985. Temporary relocation: Is it stressful to your patients? *Journal of Gerontological Nursing* 11(10):28-31.

Ethridge, P. and Lamb, G.S. 1989. Professional nursing case management improves quality, access, and costs. *Nursing Management* 20(3):30-35.

Evans, L. 1987. Sundown syndrome in institutionalized elderly. *Journal of the American Geriatrics Society* 35(2):101-108.

Faherty, B.S. and Grier, M.G. 1984. Analgesic medication for elderly people postsurgery. *Nursing Research* 33(6):369-372.

Fakouri, C. and Jones, P. 1987. Relaxation treatment: Slow stroke back rub. *Journal of Gerontological Nursing* 13(2):32-35.

Farnsworth, J. 1988. The influence of self-esteem on the subjective well-being of older divorced and widowed adults. *Dissertation Abstracts* 48(9):2603B.

Farran, C. and McCann, J. 1989. Longitudinal analysis of hope in community-based older adults. *Archives of Psychiatric Nursing* 3(5):272-276.

Farran, C. and Popovich, J. 1990. Hope: A relevant concept for geriatric psychiatry. *Archives of Psychiatric Nursing* 4(2):124-130.

Farran, C.; Salloway, J.; and Clark, D. 1990. Measurement of hope in a community-based older population. *Western Journal of Nursing Research* 12(1):42-59.

Federal Council on the Aging, U.S. Department of Health and Human Services. 1981. *The need for long-term care.* Washington D.C.: Pub. No. 81-20704.

Feldman, R.; Weiss, E.; and Small, N. 1989. Home care support program for frail elderly clients. *Applied Nursing Research* 2(1):48-49.

Ferrans, C.E.; Powers, M.J.; and Kasch, C.R. 1987. Satisfaction with health care of hemodialysis patients. *Research in Nursing and Health* 10(6):367-374.

Fishman, S. 1989. An investigation of the relationships among an older adult's life review, ego integrity, and death anxiety. *Dissertation Abstracts* 49(8):3103B.

Fitzgerald, J.; Moore, P.; and Dittus, R. 1988. The care of elderly patients with hip fractures: Changes since implementation of the prospective payment system. *The New England Journal of Medicine* November:1392-1397.

Flynn, K.T.; Norton, L.C.; and Fisher, R.L. 1987. Enternal tube feeding: Indications, practices, and outcomes. *Image: The Journal of Nursing Scholarship* 19:16-19.

Flynn, M.K. and Frantz, R. 1987. Coronary artery bypass surgery: Quality of life during early convalescence. *Heart and Lung* 16:159-167.

Flynn, R. 1986. The relationship of self-actualization, internal locus of control, and sexual activity to the experience of life satisfaction in elderly men. *Dissertation Abstracts* 46:2611B-2621.

Folden, S. 1990. On the inside looking out: Perceptions of the home bound. *Journal of Gerontological Nursing* 16(1):15-19.

Folta, A.; Metzger, B.; and Therrien, B. 1989. Pre-existing physical activity levels and cardiovascular responses across the Valsalva maneuver. *Nursing Research* 38(3):139-143.

Folta, A.; Storm, D.; and Therrien, B. 1987. The effect of aging on the intensity of cardiovascular responses during the Valsalva maneuver in healthy adults. *Heart and Lung* 16(3):330-331.

Foreman, M. 1987. Reliability and validity of mental status questionnaires in elderly hospitalized patients. *Nursing Research* 36(4):217-220.

————. 1989. Confusion in the hospitalized elderly: Incidence, onset, and associated factors. *Research in Nursing and Health* 12:21-29.

Forsyth, G.L.; Delaney, K.D.; and Gresham, M.L. 1984. Vying for a winning position: Management style of the chronically ill. *Research in Nursing and Health* 7(3):181-188.

Foster, M.F. 1987. The study of relationships among perceived current health, health promoting activities, and life satisfaction in older black adults. *Dissertation Abstracts* 48(5):1301B.

Francis, G. and Baly, A. 1986. Plush animals: Do they make a difference? *Geriatric Nursing* 7(3):140-142.

Frank, J. 1985. The effects of music therapy and guided visual imagery on chemotherapy-induced nausea and vomiting. *Oncology Nursing Forum* 12(5):47-52.

Frank-Stromborg, M. 1988. Single instruments for measuring quality of life. In *Instruments for clinical nursing research,* ed. M. Frank-Stromborg, pp. 779-795. Norwalk, Conn.: Appleton & Lange.

Frantz, R.A. and Kinney, C.K. 1986. Variables associated with skin dryness in the elderly. *Nursing Research* 35(2):98-100.

Fuller, S.S. and Larson, S.B. 1980. Life events, emotional support, and health of older people. *Research in Nursing and Health* 3(2):81-89.

Fulmer, T. and Ashley, J. 1989. Clinical indicators of elder neglect. *Applied Nursing Research* 2:161-167.

Furukawa, C. 1981. Adult health care conference: Community-oriented health maintenance for the elderly. *The Journal of Aging and Health Promotion:*105-121.

Gamroth, S.L. 1988. Long-term care resource requirements before and after the prospective payment system. *Image: The Journal of Nursing Scholarship* 20(1):7-11.

Gasper, P.M. 1988. Fluid intake: What determines how much patients drink? *Geriatric Nursing* 9(4):221-224.

Gass, K.A. 1987a. Coping strategies of widows. *Journal of Gerontological Nursing* 13(8):29-33.

———. 1987b. The health of conjugally bereaved older widows: The role of appraisal, coping, and resources. *Research in Nursing and Health* 19(1):39-47.

———. 1988. Aged widows and widowers: Similarities and differences in appraisal, coping, resources, type of death, and health dysfunction. *Archives of Psychiatric Nursing* 2(4):200-210.

Gass, K.A. and Chang, A.S. 1989. Appraisals of bereavement, coping resources, and psychosocial health dysfunction in widows and widowers. *Nursing Research* 38(1):31-36.

Gaynor, S. 1989. When the care giver becomes the patient. *Geriatric Nursing* 10(3):120-125.

Gilson, P. and Coats, S. 1980. A study of morale in low income blacks. *Journal of Gerontological Nursing* 6(7):385-388.

Given, B.; King, S.; Collins, C.; and Given, C. 1988. Family caregivers of the elderly: Involvement and reactions to care. *Archives of Psychiatric Nursing* 2(5):281-288.

Given, B.; Stommel, M.; Collins, C.; King, S.; and Given, C. 1990. Responses of elderly spouse caregivers. *Research in Nursing and Health* 13(2):77-85.

Glasspoole, L. and Aman, M. 1990. Knowledge, attitudes, and happiness of nurses working with gerontological patients. *Journal of Gerontological Nursing* 16(2):11-14.

Goldberg, W. and Fitzpatrick, J. 1980. Movement therapy with the aged. *Nursing Research* 29(6):339-346.

Gomez, G.E.; Otto, D.; Blattstein, A.; and Gomez, E.A. 1985. Beginning nursing students can change attitudes about the aged. *Journal of Gerontological Nursing* 11(1):6-11.

Goodman, J.J. 1989. Pulmonary rehabilitation and compliance with health care recommendations in chronic bronchitis and emphysema patients. *Dissertation Abstracts* 49(8):3103B.

Gorenberg, B.D. 1986. Health maintenance of the frail elderly: Informal and formal help at home. *Dissertation Abstracts* 47(1):132-133B.

Goto, L. and Braun, C. 1987. Nursing home without walls. *Journal of Gerontological Nursing* 13(1):7-9.

Graham, R. 1989. Adult day care: How families of dementia patients respond. *Journal of Gerontological Nursing* 15(3):27-31.

Grant, R. 1982. Washable pads or disposable diapers? *Geriatric Nursing* 3(4):248.

Grau, L. and Kobner, C. 1986. Comorbidity and length of stay: A case study. *Nursing and Health Care* 7(8):427-430.

Gray, P. and Stevenson, J. 1980. Changes in verbal interaction among members of resocialization groups. *Journal of Gerontological Nursing* 6(2):86.

Greene, V. and Monahan, D. 1982. The impact of visitation on patient well-being in nursing homes. *The Gerontologist* 22(4):418-423.

Gress, L.; Hassanein, R.; and Bahr, S. R. 1981. Nocturnal behavior of selected institutionalized adults. *Journal of Gerontological Nursing* 7(2):86-92.

Gross, J. 1990. Bladder dysfunction after a stroke: It's not always inevitable. *Journal of Gerontological Nursing* 16(4):20-25.

Gueldner, S. and Spradley, J. 1988. Outdoor walking lowers fatigue. *Journal of Gerontological Nursing* 14(10):6-12.

Gustafson, D.; Fiss, C.; Frayback, J.; Smelser, P.; and Hiles, M. 1980. Measuring the quality of care in nursing homes: A pilot study in Wisconsin. *Public Health Reports* 95(4):336-343.

Haeker, S. 1985. Disposable versus reusable incontinence products. *Geriatric Nursing* 6(6):345-347.

Haff, J.; McGowan, C.; Potts, C.; and Streekstra, C. 1988. Evaluating primary nursing in long-term care: Provider and consumer opinions. *Journal of Nursing Quality Assurance* 2(3):44-53.

Hain, M.J. and Chen, S.C. 1986. Health needs of the elderly. *Nursing Research* 25(6):433-439.

Hamilton, G. 1985. The roles of pet and music therapy in providing sensory stimulation to institutionalized elderly persons. *Dissertation Abstracts* 46(4): 1059-1060A.

Hamilton, J. 1989. Comfort and the hospitalized chronically ill. *Journal of Gerontological Nursing* 15(4):28-33.

Hanley, I.G. 1981. The use of signposts and active training to modify ward disorientation in elderly patients. *Journal of Behavioral Therapy and Experimental Psychiatry* 12(3):241-247.

Hargrove-Huttle, R. 1989. Virginia Henderson's nature of nursing theory and quality of life for the older adult. *Dissertation Abstracts* 49(8):3104B.

Harper, D. 1984. Application of Orem's theoretical constructs to self-care medication behaviors in the elderly. *Advances in Nursing Science* 6(3):29-46.

Harrell, J.; McConnell, E.; Wildman, D.; and Samsa, G. 1989. Do nursing diagnoses affect functional status? *Journal of Gerontological Nursing* 15(10):13-19.

Harris, M.D. 1988. The changing scene in community health nursing. *Nursing Clinics of North America* 23(3):559-568.

Harron, J. and Schaeffer, J. 1986. DRGs in the intensity of skilled nursing. *Geriatric Nursing* 7(1):31-33.

Hart, M.A. and Sliefert, M.K. 1983. Monitoring patient incidents in a long-term care facility. *Quality Review Bulletin* 9(12):356-365.

Hathaway, D. 1986. Effect of pre-operative instruction on postoperative outcomes: A meta-analysis. *Nursing Research* 35(5):269-275.

Haviland, S. and Garlinghouse, C. 1985. Nursing foot clinics fulfill a great need. *Geriatric Nursing* 6(6):338-341.

Hayter, J. 1983. Sleep behaviors of older persons. *Nursing Research* 32(4):242-246.

Heater, B.; Becker, A.; and Olson, R. 1988. Nursing interventions and patient outcomes: A meta-analysis of studies. *Nursing Research* 37(5):303-307.

Heidenreich, T. and Giuffre, M. 1990. Postoperative temperature measurement. *Nursing Research* 39(3):153-155.

Hendrich, A. 1988. An effective unit-based fall prevention plan. *Journal of Nursing Quality Assurance* 3(1):28-36.

Hernandez, M. and Miller, J. 1986. How to reduce falls. *Geriatric Nursing* 7(2):97-102.

Herth, K. 1990. Relationship of hope, coping styles, concurrent losses and setting to grief resolution in the elderly widow(er). *Research in Nursing and Health* 13(2):109-117.

Hess, P. 1986. Chinese and Hispanic elders and OTC drugs. *Geriatric Nursing* 7(6):314-318.

Hewitt, S.M.; LeSage, J.; Roberts, K.L.; and Ellor, J.R. 1985. Process auditing in long-term care facilities. *Quality Review Bulletin* 11(1):6-16.

Higgins, P. 1983. Can 98.6°F be a fever in disguise? *Geriatric Nursing* 4(2):101-102.

Hilbert, Gail A. 1985. Spouse support and myocardial infarction patient compliance. *Nursing Research* 34(4):217-220.

Hobler, K.E. and Howlett, P.A. 1985. Surgery in the very elderly. *Quality Review Bulletin* 11(11):339-341.

Hoeffer, B. 1987a. A causal model of loneliness among older single women. *Archives of Psychiatric Nursing* 1(5):366-373.

————. 1987b. Predictors of life outlook of older single women. *Research in Nursing and Health* 10(2):111-117.

Hogan, A.J. and Smith, D.W. 1987. Patient classification and resource allocation in Veterans Administration nursing homes. *Advances in Nursing Science* 9(3):56-71.

Hogstel, M.D. 1979. Use of reality orientation with aging confused patients. *Nursing Research* 28(3):161-165.

Horgan, P. 1987. Health status perceptions affect health-related behaviors. *Journal of Gerontological Nursing* 13(12):30-33.

Howe, M.; Coulton, M.; Almon, G.; and Sandrick, K. 1980a. Developing scaled outcome criteria for a target patient population. *Quality Review Bulletin* 6(3):17-23.

————. 1980b. Use of scaled outcome criteria for a target patient population. *Quality Review Bulletin* 6(4):15-21.

Hu, T.; Kaltreider, D.; and Igou, J. 1989. Incontinence products: Which is best? *Geriatric Nursing* 10(4):184-186.

————. 1990. The cost-effectiveness of disposable versus reusable diapers: A controlled experiment in a nursing home. *Journal of Gerontological Nursing* 16(2):19-24.

Hughston, G. and Merriam, S. 1982. Reminiscence: A nonformal technique for improving cognitive functioning in the aged. *International Journal of Aging and Human Development* 15(2):139-149.

Humphreys, D.; Mason, R.; Guthrie, M.; Liem, C.; and Stern, E. 1988. The Miami channeling program: Case management and cost control. *Quality Review Bulletin* 14(5):154-160.

Huss, J.; Buckwalter, K.; and Stolley, J. 1988. Nursing's impact on life satisfaction. *Journal of Gerontological Nursing* 14(5):31-36.

Hussian, R.A. and Brown, D.C. 1987. Use of two-dimensional grid patterns to limit hazardous ambulation in demented patients. *Journal of Gerontology* 42(5):558-560.

Hyland, D. and Kirkland, V.J. 1980. Infrared therapy for skin ulcers. *American Journal of Nursing* 80(10):1800-1801.

Igou, J.; Hawkins, J.; Johnson, E.; and Utley, Q. 1989. Nurse-managed approach to care. *Geriatric Nursing* 10(1):32-34.

Innes, E.M. 1985. Maintaining fall prevention. *Quality Review Bulletin* 11(7):217-221.

Innes, E.M. and Turman, W.G. 1983. Evaluation of patient falls. *Quality Review Bulletin* 9(2):30-35.

Jacox, A. 1987. The OTA report: A policy analysis. *Nursing Outlook* 35(6):262-267.

Jamieson, M. 1990. Block nursing: Practicing autonomous professional nursing in the community. *Nursing and Health Care* 11(5):250-263.

Jamieson, M.; Campbell, J.; and Clarke, S. 1989. The block nurse program. *The Gerontologist* 29(1):124-127.

Janken, J.K.; Reynolds, B.A.; and Swiech, K. 1986. Patient falls in the acute care setting: Identifying risk factors. *Nursing Research* 35(4):215-219.

Janssen, J. and Giberson, D. 1988. Remotivation therapy. *Journal of Gerontological Nursing* 14(6):31-34.

Jezierski, M. 1988. Minneapolis pre-hospital do-not-resuscitate form. *Journal of Emergency Nursing* 14(4):26-29A.

Johnson, B.K. 1987. The sexual interest, participation, and satisfaction of older men and women. *Dissertation Abstracts* 47(12):4824B.

Johnson, F.; Cloyd, C.; and Wer, J. 1982. Life satisfaction of poor urban black aged. *Advances in Nursing Science* 4(3):27-35.

Johnson, F.L.; Foxall, M.J.; Kidwell-Udin, M.A.; Miller, G.; and Stolzer, M.E. 1984. Life satisfaction in the minority elderly. *Issues in Mental Health Nursing* 6(1-2):189-207.

Johnson, J. 1987. Selecting nursing activities for hospitalized clients. *Journal of Gerontological Nursing* 13(10):29-33.

Johnson, J. and Moore, J. 1988. The drug taking practices in the rural elderly. *Applied Nursing Research* 1(3):128-131.

Johnson, M. and Maguire, M. 1989. Give me a break: Benefits of a caregiver support service. *Journal of Gerontological Nursing* 15(11):22-26.

Johnson, M. and Werner, C. 1982. We had no choice: A study in familial guilt feelings surrounding nursing home care. *Journal of Gerontological Nursing* 8(11):641-654.

Johnston, J. E. 1987. Fall prevention responses in the elderly. *Dissertation Abstracts* 48(4):1004B.

————. 1988. The elderly and fall prevention. *Applied Nursing Research* 1(3):140.

Johnston, L. and Gueldner, S. 1989. Using mnemonics to boost memory in the elderly. *Journal of Gerontological Nursing* 15(8):22-26.

Jones, M. 1985. Patient violence: Report of 200 incidents. *Journal of Psychosocial Nursing* 23(6):12-17.

Jordan-Marsh, M. and Neutra, R. 1985. Relationship of health locus of control and lifestyle change programs. *Research in Nursing and Health* 8(1):3-11.

Justin, R.G. and Johnson, R.A. 1989. Recording end-of-life directives on hospital admission. *Nursing Management* 20(3):65-68.

Kalayjian, A. 1989. Coping with cancer: The spouse's perspective. *Archives of Psychiatric Nursing* 3(3):166-172.

Kaltreider, D.; Hu, T.; Igou, J.; Yu, L.; and Craighead, W. 1990. Can reminders curb incontinence? *Geriatric Nursing* 11(1):17-19.

Kaplan, S.W. 1988. An investigation of day care facilities for care of the moderately to severely demented older adults. *Dissertation Abstracts* 49(6):2129B.

Karl, C. 1982. The effect of an exercise program on self-care activities for the institutionalized elderly. *Journal of Gerontological Nursing* 8(5):282-285.

Kartman, L. 1977. The use of music as a program tool with regressed geriatric patients. *Journal of Gerontological Nursing* 3(4):38-42.

Keane, S. and Sells, S. 1990. Recognizing depression in the elderly. *Journal of Gerontological Nursing* 16(1):21-25.

Keenan, R.; Redshaw, A.; Munson, J.; and Mundt, W. 1983. The benefits of a drug holiday. *Geriatric Nursing* 4(2):103-104.

Keller, M.; Levinthal, H.; Prohaska, T.; and Linthal, E. 1989. Beliefs about aging and illness in a community sample. *Research in Nursing and Health* 12(4):247-255.

Kelly-Hayes, M. 1987. Quality of survivorship following stroke: Cognitive, physical, and social factors. *Dissertation Abstracts* 48(4):1004B.

Kim, K.K. 1986. Response time and health care learning of elderly patients. *Research in Nursing and Health* 9(3):233-239.

King, F.E.; Figge, J.; and Harman, P. 1986. The elderly coping at home: A study of continuity of nursing care. *Journal of Advanced Nursing* 11:41-46.

King, K.; Dimond, M.; and McCance, K. 1987. Coping with relocation. *Geriatric Nursing* 8(5):258-261.

King, K.B.; Norsen, L.H.; Robertson, R.K.; and Hicks, G. L. 1987. Patient management of pain medication after cardiac surgery. *Nursing Research* 36(3):145-150.

Kirschling, J.M. and Austin, J.K. 1988. Assessing support: The recently widowed. *Archives of Psychiatric Nursing* 2(2):81-86.

Kline, N.W. 1989. Psychophysiological processes of stress in people with a chronic physical illness. *Dissertation Abstracts* 49(6):2129B.

Knaus, W.A.; Draper, E.A.; Wagner, D.P.; and Zimmerman, J.E. 1986. Evaluation of outcomes from intensive care in major medical centers. *Annals of Internal Medicine* 104:410-418.

Kobza, L.L. 1983. Assessing postmastectomy care in a community hospital. *Quality Review Bulletin* 9(4):116-119.

Kolanowski, A. and Gunter, L. 1981. Hypothermia in the elderly. *Geriatric Nursing* 2(5):362-365.

Kongable, L.; Buckwalter, K.; and Stolley, J. 1989. The effects of pet therapy on the social behavior of institutionalized Alzheimer's clients. *Archives of Psychiatric Nursing* 3(4):191-198.

Kovner, C.T. 1986. Relationship of nurse-patient agreement on importance of outcomes to patient satisfaction and length of stay. *Dissertation Abstracts* 46:2624B.

Krommings, S.K. and Ostwald, S.K. 1987. The public health nurse as a discharge planner: Patients' perceptions of the discharge process. *Public Health Nursing* 4:224-229.

Kutlenios, R.M. 1985. A comparison of holistic, mental, and physical health nursing interventions with the elderly. *Dissertation Abstracts* 46:995B.

L'abbe, K.A.; Detsky, A.S.; and O'Rourke, K. 1987. Meta-analysis in clinical research. *Annals of Internal Medicine* 107:214-233.

Labi, M.; Phillips, T.; and Gresham, G. 1980. Psychosocial disability in physically restored long-term stroke survivors. *Archives of Physical Medicine Rehabilitation* 61:561-565.

Laborde, J.M. and Powers, M.J. 1985. Life satisfaction, health control orientation, and illness-related factors in persons with osteoarthritis. *Research in Nursing and Health* 8(2):183-190.

Lacey, A.L. 1989. Health beliefs and health behavior in elderly, chronically ill males. *Dissertation Abstracts* 49(8):3106B.

LaLonde, B. 1987. The general symptom distress scale: A home care outcome measure. *Quality Review Bulletin* 13(7):243-250.

Lambert, V.A. 1985. Study of factors associated with psychological well-being in rheumatoid arthritic women. *Image: The Journal of Nursing Scholarship* 17:50-53.

Lamont, C.T.; Sampson, S.; Matthias, R.; and Kane, R. 1983. The outcome of hospitalization for acute illness in the elderly. *Journal of the American Geriatrics Society* 31:282-288.

Lang, N.M. 1980. *Nurse Planning Series Volume 12, Quality Assurance in Nursing: A Selected Bibliography.* Washington, D.C.: U.S. Government Printing Office.

Lang, N.M. and Clinton, J. 1984. Assessment of quality of nursing care. In *Annual review of nursing research,* vol. 2, ed. H. Werley and J. Fitzpatrick, pp. 135-163. New York: Springer.

Langland, R. and Panicucci, C. 1983. Effects of touch on communication with elderly confused clients. *Journal of Gerontological Nursing* 8(3):152-155.

Lantz, J. 1985. In search of agents for self-care. *Journal of Gerontological Nursing* 11(7):10-13.

Lappe, J.M. 1987. Reminiscing: The life review therapy. *Journal of Gerontological Nursing* 13(4):12-16.

Lara, L.; Troop, P.; and Beadleson-Baird, M. 1990. Risk of urinary tract infection in bowel incontinent men. *Journal of Gerontological Nursing* 16(5):14-26.

Larson, J.L. 1986. Inspiratory muscle training in patients with COPD. *Dissertation Abstracts* 47(1):133B.

Lashley, M.E. 1987. Predictors of breast self-examination practice among elderly women. *Advances in Nursing Science* 9(4):25-34.

Lauton, M.P.; Moss, M.; and Moles, E. 1984. Pet ownership: A research note. *The Gerontologist* 24(2):208-210.

Leja, A. 1989. Using guided imagery to combat postsurgical depression. *Journal of Gerontological Nursing* 15(4):6-11.

LeSage, J.; Slimmer, L.; Lopez, M.; and Ellor, J. 1989. Learned helplessness. *Journal of Gerontological Nursing* 15(5):16-23.

Leslie, F. 1981. Nursing diagnosis: Use in long-term care. *American Journal of Nursing* 81(5):1012-1014.

Lewandowski, W.; Daly, B.; McClish, D.K.; Juknialis, B.W.; and Younger, S.J. 1985. Treatment and care of "do not resuscitate" patients in a medical intensive careunit. *Heart and Lung* 14:175-181.

Lewis, M.A.; Kane, R.L.; Kretin, S.; and Clark, V. 1985. The immediate and subsequent outcomes of nursing home care. *American Journal of Public Health* 75(7):758-762.

Lincoln, R. 1984. What do nurses know about confusion in the aged? *Journal of Gerontological Nursing* 10(8):26-32.

Linn, M.W.; Gurel, L.; and Linn, B.S. 1977. Patient outcome as a measure of quality of nursing home care. *American Journal of Public Health* 67(4):337-344.

Llewellyn, J.; Martin, B.; Shekleton, M.; and Firlit, S. 1988. Analysis of falls in the acute surgical and cardiovascular surgical patient. *Applied Nursing Research* 1(3):116-121.

Long, M.L. 1985. Incontinence. *Journal of Gerontological Nursing* 11(1):30-41.

Longman, A. and DeWalt, E. 1986. A guide for oral assessment. *Geriatric Nursing* 7(5):252-253.

Louis, M. 1981. Personal space boundary needs of elderly persons: An empirical study. *Journal of Gerontological Nursing* 7(7):395-400.

Loveridge, K. and Heineken, J. 1988. Confirming interactions. *Journal of Gerontological Nursing* 14(5):27-30.

Lund, D.; Feinhauer, L.; and Miller, J. 1985. Living together: Grandparents and children tell their problems. *Journal of Gerontological Nursing* 11(11):29-33.

Lund, D.; Johnson, R.; Baraki, H.; and Dimond, M. 1984. Can pets help the bereaved? *Journal of Gerontological Nursing* 10(6):8-12.

Maas, M.D. and Buckwalter, K. 1988. A special Alzheimer's unit: Phase I baseline data. *Applied Nursing Research* 1(1):41.

Macauley, C.; Murray, L.; and Ellis, H. 1980. Patient-administered drugs in a municipal hospital. *Geriatric Nursing* 1(2):109-111.

Maddox, M. 1990. Is there a link between dementia and phenylketonuria? *Journal of Gerontological Nursing* 16(5):18-23.

Magilvy, J. 1985. Quality of life of hearing-impaired older women. *Nursing Research* 34(3):140-144.

Magilvy, J.; Brown, N.; and Dydyn, J. 1988. The experience of home health care: Perceptions of older adults. *Public Health Nursing* 5(3):140-145.

Magnani, L.I. 1986. The relationship of hardiness and self-perceived health to activity in groups of independently functioning older adults. *Dissertation Abstracts* 46(12):4184B.

Mahoney, E.K. 1985. The interaction of physical illness, coping focus, and perceived social support and their relationship to recovery from stroke. *Dissertation Abstracts* 47(5):1929B.

Marchette, L. and Holloman, F. 1986. Length of stay: Significant variables. *Journal of Nursing Administration* 16(3):12-20.

Mason, D.J. 1987. Circadian body temperature and activation rhythms and well-being of independent older women. *Dissertation Abstracts* 48(6).1641B.

Matheson, M. and McConnell, E. 1988. *Gerontological nursing concepts and practice.* Philadelphia: J.B. Saunders.

Matthiesen, V. 1989. Guilt and grief when daughters place mothers in nursing homes. *Journal of Gerontological Nursing* 15(7):11-15.

Mayers, K. and Griffin, M. 1990. The play project: Use of stimulus objects with demented patients. *Journal of Gerontological Nursing* 16(1):32-37.

McCann, J.J. 1988. Long-term home care for the elderly: Perceptions of nurses, physicians, and primary caregivers. *Quality Review Bulletin* 14(3):66-74.

McCracken, A. 1987. Emotional impact of possession loss. *Journal of Gerontological Nursing* 13(2):14-19.

McCracken, A. and Fitzwater, E. 1989. The right environment for Alzheimer's. *Geriatric Nursing* 10(6):293-294.

McDaniel, R.W. 1987. Relationship of participation in health promotion behaviors to quality of life. *Dissertation Abstracts* 48(7):1040B.

McGovern, K. and Newbern, V. 1988. Long-term care facility: DRG impact. *Journal of Gerontological Nursing* 14(9):17-20.

McMillan, B.A. and Jasmund, J.M. 1985. A quality assurance study of height and weight measurement. *Quality Review Bulletin* 11(2):53-56.

McPhee, S.J.; Frank, D.H.; Lewis, C.; Bush, D.E.; and Smith, C.R. 1983. Influence of "discharge interview" on patient knowledge, compliance, and functional status after hospitalization. *Medical Care* 21:755-767.

Mech, A.B. 1980. Evaluating the process of nursing care in long-term care facilities. *Quarterly Review Bulletin* 6(3):24-30.

Melillo, K. 1980. Informal activity involvement and the perceived rate of time passage for an older institutionalized population. *Journal of Gerontological Nursing* 6(7):392.

Meyer, P.A. 1987. Nursing home residents' water intake. *Dissertation Abstracts* 47(3):996B.

Mezey, M.; Lynaugh, J.; and Cherry, J. 1984. The teaching nursing home program. *Nursing Outlook* 32(3):146-150.

Michaelsson, E.; Norberg, A.; and Norberg, B. 1987. Feeding methods for demented patients in end stage of life. *Geriatric Nursing* 8(2)69-73.

Micheletti, J.A. and Shlala, T.J. 1986. RUGS II: Implications for management and quality in long term care. *Quality Review Bulletin* 12(7):235-242.

Miller, J. 1990. Assessing urinary incontinence. *Journal of Gerontological Nursing* 16(3):15-19.

Miller, S.P. and Russel, D. 1980. Elements promoting satisfaction as identified by residents in the nursing home. *Journal of Gerontological Nursing* 6(3):121.

Mills, R. 1986. The relationship of interpersonal time, life position, and stroking to life satisfaction of older individuals. *Dissertation Abstracts* 46:2625B.

Mion, L.; Frengley, J.D. and Adams, M. 1986. Nursing patients 75 years and older. *Nursing Management* 17(9):24-28.

Mohide, E.A.; Tugwell, P.; Caulfield, P.; Chambers, L.; Dunnett, C.; Baptiste, S.; Byne,R.; Patterson, C.; Rudnick, V.; and Pill, M. 1988. A randomized trial of quality assurance in nursing homes. *Medical Care* 26(6):554-556.

Morse, J.; Dixon, H.; and Tylko, S. 1985. The patient who falls...and falls again: Defining the aged at risk. *Journal of Gerontological Nursing* 11(11):15-18.

Moyer, N.C. 1987. Outcomes after termination of Medicare home health services: Their relationship to the resources and well-being of elderly caregiving spouses. *Dissertation Abstracts* 47:2840B.

Mulcahy, N. and Rosa, N. 1981. Reality orientation in a general hospital. *Geriatric Nursing* 2(4):264-268.

Mumma, N.L. 1987. Quality and cost control of home care services through coordinated funding. *Quality Review Bulletin* 13(8):271-278.

Munro, B.; Brown, L.; and Heitman, B. 1989. Pressure ulcers: one bed or another? *Geriatric Nursing* 10(4):190-192.

Murray, R.; Huelskoetter, M.; and Odriscol, B. 1980. *Nursing process in late life.* Englewood Cliffs, N.J.: Prentice-Hall.

Nagley, S.J. 1986. Predicting and preventing confusion in your patients. *Journal of Gerontological Nursing* 12(3):27-31.

Naylor, M. 1990. Comprehensive discharge planning for the hospitalized elderly: A pilot study. *Nursing Research* 39(1):42-47.

Negley, E. and Manley, J. 1990. Environmental intervention in assaultive behavior. *Journal of Gerontological Nursing* 16(3):29-33.

Neildinger, S.H.; Scroggins, K.; and Kennedy, L.M. 1987. Cost evaluation of discharge planning for hospitalized elderly. *Nursing Economic$* 5:225-230.

Nelson, P. 1989. Ethnic differences in intrinsic/extrinsic religious orientation and depression in the elderly. *Archives of Psychiatric Nursing* 3(4):199-204.

———. 1990. Intrinsic/extrinsic religious orientation of the elderly: Relationship to depression and self-esteem. *Journal of Gerontological Nursing* 16(2):29-35.

Neubauer, J.; LeSage, J.; and Roberts, C. 1989. Making the family a partner in quality assurance. *Geriatric Nursing* 10(1):35-37.

Newman, M.A. and Gaudiano, J.K. 1984. Depression as an explanation for decreased subjective time in the elderly. *Nursing Research* 33(3):137-139.

Niemoller, J. 1990. Change of pace for Alzheimer's patients. *Geriatric Nursing* 11(2):86-87.

Nodhturft, V.L. and Sweeney, N.M. 1982. Reality orientation therapy for the institutionalized elderly. *Journal of Gerontological Nursing* 8(7):396-401.

Nosek, L.J. 1987. Explanation of hospital stay by nursing diagnoses, medical diagnoses, and social position. *Dissertation Abstracts* 47(7)2840B.

Oberst, M.T.; Graham, D.; Geller, N.L.; Maus, W.; Stearns, M.W., Jr.; and Tiernan, E. 1981. Catheter management programs and postoperative urinary dysfunction. *Research in Nursing and Health* 4(1):175-181.

O'Connell, K.; Hamera, E.; Kanapp, T.; Cassmeyer, V.; Eaks, G.; and Fox, M. 1984. Symptom use and self-regulation in Type 2 diabetes. *Advances in Nursing Science* 3(3):19-28.

Olson, B.K. 1984. Player piano music as therapy for the elderly. *Journal of Music Therapy* 21(1):35-45.

Oudt, B.M. 1989. Self-reported health status and health behaviors of women aged 85 years and older. *Dissertation Abstracts* 49(7):2569B.

Ouslander, J.G.; Morishita, L.; Blaustein, J.; Orzeck, S.; Dunn, S.; and Sayre, J. 1987. Clinical, functional, and psychosocial characteristics of an incontinent nursing home population. *Journal of Gerontology* 42(6):631-637.

Pacini, C. and Fitzpatrick, J. 1982. Sleep patterns of hospitalized and nonhospitalizedaged individuals. *Journal of Gerontological Nursing* 8(6):327-332.

Packard, J. 1988. Health care system dependency among older adults: Patterns of hospital use by lung cancer patients. *Dissertation Abstracts* 48(2):363B.

Padilla, G.V. and Grant, M.M. 1985. Quality of life as a cancer nursing outcome variable. *Advances in Nursing Science* 8(1):15-24.

Pajk, M.; Craven, G.A.; Cameron, J.; Shipps, T.; and Bennum, N.W. 1986. Investigating the problem of pressure sores. *Journal of Gerontological Nursing* 12(7):11-16.

Palmateer, L.M. and McCartney, J.R. 1985. Do nurses know when patients have cognitive deficits? *Journal of Gerontological Nursing* 11(2):6-16.

Palmer, M.; McCormick, K.; and Langord, A. 1989. Do nurses consistently document incontinence? *Journal of Gerontological Nursing* 15(12):11-16.

Panniers, T.L. and Newlander, J. 1986. The adverse patient occurrences inventory: Validity, reliability, and implications. *Quality Review Bulletin* 12(9):311-315.

Panniers, T.L. and Tomkiewicz, Z.M. 1985. The ICD-9-CM DRGs: Increased homogeneity through use of AS-SCORE. *Quality Review Bulletin* 11(2):47-52.

Parent, C. and Wahll, A. 1984. Are physical activity, self-esteem, and depression related? *Journal of Gerontological Nursing* 10(9):8-10.

Parsons, W. 1984. Reminiscence group therapy with older persons: A field experiment. *Dissertation Abstracts* 45(4):1040-1041A.

Pascucci, M.A. 1988. Health values, incentives, and social support related to health promotion behaviors in the well elderly. *Dissertation Abstracts* 46(4):1006B.

Pasquale, D.K. 1987. A basis for prospective payment for home care. *Image: The Journal of Nursing Scholarship* 19:186-191.

Patsdaughter, C. and Pesznecker, B. 1988. Medication regimes in the elderly home care client. *Journal of Gerontological Nursing* 14(10):30-34.

Pearson, B.D. and Droessler, D. 1988. Continence through nursing care. *Geriatric Nursing* 9(6):347-349.

Pender, N.J. 1985. Effects of progressive muscle relaxation training on anxiety and health locus of control among hypertensive adults. *Research in Nursing and Health* 8(1):67-72.

Pensiero, M. and Adams, M. 1987. Dress and self-esteem. *Journal of Gerontological Nursing* 13(10):11-17.

Perrotta, P. and Meacham, J. 1981-82. Can reminiscing intervention alter depression and self-esteem? *International Journal of Aging and Human Development* 14(1):23-30.

Perry, J. 1981. Effectiveness of teaching in the rehabilitation of patients with chronic bronchitis and emphysema. *Nursing Research* 30(4):219-228.

Petrou, M. and Obenchain, J. 1987. Reducing incidence of illness post-transfer. *Geriatric Nursing* 8(5):264-266.

Petrucci, C.; McCormick, C.; and Scheve, A. 1987. Documenting patient care needs: Do nurses do it? *Journal of Gerontological Nursing* 13(11):34-38.

Phillips, L.R. and Rempusheski, V.F. 1985. A decision-making model for diagnosing and intervening in elder abuse and neglect. *Nursing Research* 34(3):134-139.

———. 1986. Caring for the frail elderly at home: Toward a theoretical explanation of the dynamics of poor quality family care giving. *Advances in Nursing Science* 8(4):62-84.

Pohl, J.M. and Fuller, S.S. 1980. Perceived choice, social interaction, and dimensions of morale of residents in a home for the aged. *Research in Nursing and Health* 3(4):147-157.

Polyneaux, R.; Papciak, B.; and Woem, D. 1987. Coagulation studies and the indwelling heparinized catheter. *Heart and Lung* 16(1):20-23.

Powers, B.A. 1988. Social network, social support in elderly institutionalized people. *Advances in Nursing Science* 10(2):40-58.

Poznanski, C. 1987. Types and meanings of caring behaviors among elderly nursing home residents. *Dissertation Abstracts* 48(6):1643B.

Preston, D. and Dellasega, C. 1990. Elderly women in stress: Does marriage make a difference? *Journal of Gerontological Nursing* 16(4):26-32.

Preston, D. and Grimes, J. 1987. A study in differences in social support. *Journal of Gerontological Nursing* 13(2):36-40.

Pritchard, V. 1985. Watch out! Urinary tract infections must not spread. *Journal of Gerontological Nursing* 11(5):16-19.

———. 1988. Tube feeding related pneumonias. *Journal of Gerontological Nursing* 14(7):32-36.

Rainville, N.G. 1984. Effect of an implemented fall prevention program on the frequency of patient falls. *Quality Review Bulletin* 10(9):287-291.

Rainwater, A.J. 1988. Elderly loneliness and its relation to residential care. *Journal of Gerontological Nursing* 6(10):593-599.

Rantz, M. and Egan, K. 1987. Reducing death from translocation syndrome. *American Journal of Nursing* 87(10):1351-1352.

Rauckhorst, L. 1987. Health habits of elderly widows. *Journal of Gerontological Nursing* 13(8):19-22.

Reed, A.T. and Birge, S. 1988. Screening for osteoporosis. *Journal of Gerontological Nursing* 14(7):18-20.

Reed, P. 1989. Mental health of older adults. *Western Journal of Nursing Research* 11(2):143-163.

Reed, P.G. 1986a. Developmental resources and depression in the elderly. *Nursing Research* 35(6):368-374.

———. 1986b. Religiousness among terminally ill and healthy adults. *Research in Nursing and Health* 9(1):9, 35-41.

Reeve, W. and Ivison, D. 1985. Use of environmental manipulation and classroom and modified informal reality orientation with institutionalized, confused elderly patients. *Age and Aging* 14:119-121.

Remondet, J. and Hansson, R.O. 1987. Assessing a widow's grief: A short index. *Journal of Gerontological Nursing* 13(4):31-34.

Reynolds, M. 1989. Eliminating pressure sore risk. In *Research review: Studies for nursing practice,* ed. L. Cronenwett, p.3. Baltimore: Williams & Wilkins.

Rice, V.H.; Caldwell, M.; Butler, S.; and Robinson, J. 1986. Relaxation training and response to cardiac catheterization: A pilot study. *Nursing Research* 35(1):39-43.

Richter, J. 1987. Support: A resource during crisis of mate loss. *Journal of Gerontological Nursing* 13(11):18-22.

———. 1989. Providing nursing home care for the chronically mentally ill. *Journal of Gerontological Nursing* 15(6):18-23.

Riddick, C.C. 1985. Health, aquariums, and the noninstitutionalized elderly. In *Pets and the family,* ed. M. B. Sussman, pp.163-173. New York: Haworth Press.

Robb, S. 1985. Urinary incontinence verification in elderly men. *Nursing Research* 34(5):278-282.

Robb, S. and Stegman, C. 1983. Companion animals and elderly people: A challenge for evaluators of social support. *The Gerontologist* 23(3):277-282.

Robb, S.; Stegman, C.; and Wolanin, M.O. 1986. No research versus research with compromised results: A study of validation therapy. *Nursing Research* 35(2):113-118.

Roberts, B.L. 1989. The effects of walking on balance among elders. *Nursing Research* 38(3):180-182.

Roberts, B.L. and Lincoln, R.E. 1988. Cognitive disturbance in hospitalization and institutionalized elderly. *Research in Nursing and Health* 11(5):309-319.

Robinson, K.M. 1988. A social skills training program for adult caregivers. *Advances in Nursing Science* 10(2):59-72.

———. 1989a. Adjustment to caregiving in older wives: Variations in social support, health, and past marital adjustment. *Dissertation Abstracts* 49(7).

———. 1989b. Predictors of depression among wife caregivers' experience. *Nursing Research* 38(6):359-363.

Rodgers, B. 1989. Loneliness: Easing the pain of the hospitalized elderly. *Journal of Gerontological Nursing* 15(8):16-21.

Rosendahl, P. and Ross, V. 1982. Does your behavior affect your patient's response? *Journal of Gerontological Nursing* 8(10):572-575.

Rosswurm, M. 1989. Assessment of perceptual processing deficits in persons with Alzheimer's disease. *Western Journal of Nursing Research* 11(4):456-468.

Rubenstein, L.Z.; Rubenstein, L.V.; and Josephson, K.R. 1989. *Quality of health care for older people in America.* A report to the Institute of Medicine, February 1, 1989, Washington, D.C.

Ryden, M. 1984. Morale and perceived control in institutionalized elderly. *Nursing Research* 33(3):130-136.

Ryden, M. and Knopman, D. 1989. Assess not assume: Measuring the morale of cognitively impaired elderly. *Journal of Gerontological Nursing* 15(11):27-32.

Ryden, M.B. 1985. Environmental support for autonomy in the institutionalized elderly. *Research in Nursing and Health* 8:363-371.

Savishinsky, J. 1985. Pets and family relationships among nursing home residents. In *Pets and the family,* ed. M.B. Sussman, pp. 109-134. New York: Haworth Press.

Schafer, D. 1985. Reminiscence groups and the institutionalized elderly: An experiment. *Dissertation Abstracts* 46(4):160A.

Schafer, S. 1989. An aggressive approach to promoting health responsibility. *Journal of Gerontological Nursing* 15(4):22-27.

Schank, M. and Lough, M. 1989. Maintaining health and independence of elderly women. *Journal of Gerontological Nursing* 15(6):8-11.

Schank, M.J. and Conrad, D. 1977. A survey of the well-elderly and their foot problems, practices, and needs. *Journal of Gerontological Nursing* 3(6):10-15.

Schneider, J. 1987. Effects of caffeine ingestion on heart rate, blood pressure, mild cardio-oxygen consumption, and cardiac rhythm in acute mild cardio-infarction patients. *Heart and Lung* 16(2):167-174.

Schneille, J.; Traughper, B.; Morgan, D.; Embry, J.; Binion, A.; and Coleman, A. 1983. Management of geriatric incontinence in nursing homes. *Journal of Applied Behavioral Analysis* 16(2):235-241.

Schultz, P.R. and Magilvy, J. 1988. Assessing community health needs of the elderly population: Comparisons of three strategies. *Journal of Advanced Nursing* 13:193-202.

Schultz, P.R. and McGlone, F. 1977. Primary health care provided to the elderly by a nurse practitioner/physician team: Analysis of cost-effectiveness. *Journal of the American Geriatrics Society* 25(10):443-446.

Schwartz, D. 1980. Hamlet dweller-city dweller. *Geriatric Nursing* 1(2):128-132.

Schwartz, R.; Zaremba, M.; and Ra, K. 1985. Third-party coverage for diabetes education program. *Quality Review Bulletin* 11(7):213-216.

Schwirian, P. 1982. Life satisfaction among nursing home residents. *Geriatric Nursing* 3(2):111-117.

Scott, D.W.; Oberst, M.T.; and Bookbinder, M.I. 1984. Stress-coping response to genito-urinary carcinoma in men. *Nursing Research* 33(6):325-329.

Scura, K. and Wipple, B. 1990. Older adults as an HIV-positive risk group. *Journal of Gerontological Nursing* 16(2):6-10.

Scura, K.W. 1988. Audiological assessment program. *Journal of Gerontological Nursing* 14(10):19-25.

Seaman, L. and Roth L. 1989. Active treatment for long-term psychiatric patients. *Geriatric Nursing* 10(5):232-234.

Sellers, J.B. 1986. The influence of a confidante on the morale of institutionalized elderly women. *Dissertation Abstracts* 47(4):1492B.

Settles, H. 1985. A pilot study in reality orientation for the confused elderly. *Journal of Gerontological Nursing* 1(5):11-16.

Sexton, D.L. 1984. The supporting cast: Wives of COPD patients. *Journal of Gerontological Nursing* 10(2):82-85.

Sexton, D.L. and Munro, B.H. 1985. Impact of a husband's chronic illness (COPD) on the spouse's life. *Research in Nursing and Health* 8(1):83-90.

Shamanasky, S. and Hamilton, W. 1979. The health behavioral awareness test: Self-care education for the elderly. *Journal of Gerontological Nursing* 5(1):29-32.

Shanas, E. 1974. Health status of older people: Cross-national complications. *American Journal of Public Health* 3:261-264.

Shelley, S.I.; Zahorchak, R.M.; and Gambrill, C.D.S. 1987. Aggressiveness of nursing care for older patients and those with do-not-resuscitate orders. *Nursing Research* 36(3):157-162.

Shomaker, D. 1987. Problematic behavior in the Alzheimer's patient: Retrospection as a method of understanding and counseling. *The Gerontologist* 27(3):370-375.

Simon, J. 1990. Humor and its relationship to perceived health, life satisfaction, and morale in older adults. *Issues in Mental Health Nursing* 11(1):17-31.

Simons, J. 1985. Does incontinence affect your client's self-concept? *Journal of Gerontological Nursing* 11(6):37-40.

Slimmer, L.; Edwards-Beckett, J.; LeSage, J.; Ellor, J.; and Lopez, M. 1990. Helping those who don't help themselves. *Geriatric Nursing* 11(1):20-22.

Slimmer, L.; Lopez, M.; LeSage, J.; and Ellor, J. 1987. Perceptions of learned helplessness. *Journal of Gerontological Nursing* 13(5):33-37.

Small, N.R. and Walsh, M.B. 1988. *Teaching nursing homes: The nursing perspective.* Owings Mills, Md.: National Health Publishing.

Smallegan, M. 1981. Decision making for nursing home admission: A preliminary study. *Journal of Gerontological Nursing* 7(5):280-285.

————. 1985. There was nothing else to do: Needs for care before nursing home admission. *The Gerontologist* 25(4):364-369.

Sovie, M.D. 1989. Clinical nursing practices and patient outcomes: Evaluation, evolution, and revolution. *Nursing Economic$* 7(2):79-85.

Sowell, V.A.; Schnelle, J.F.; Hu, T.; and Traughber, B. 1987. A cost comparison of five methods of managing urinary incontinence. *Quality Review Bulletin* 13(12):411-414.

Speake, D.; Cowart, M.; and Pellet, K. 1989. Health perceptions and life styles of the elderly. *Research in Nursing and Health* 12(2):93-100.

Spellbring, A.; Gannon, M.; Kleckner, T.; and Conway, K. 1988. Improving safety for hospitalized elderly. *Journal of Gerontological Nursing* 14(2):31-37.

Spitzer, M.E. 1988. Taste acuity in institutionalized and noninstitutionalized elderly men. *Journal of Gerontology* 43(3):71-74.

Spitzer, W.; Dobston, A.; Hall, J.; Chesterman, E.; Levi, J.; and Shepherd, R. 1981. Measuring the quality of life of cancer patients: A concise QL-index for use by physicians. *Journal of Chronic Disease* 34(12):585-597.

Stanley, M.J. 1988. Correlates of activity levels for individuals between the ages of 60 and 75 with cardiac disease who have completed a structured cardiac rehabilitation program. *Dissertation Abstracts* 49(6).

Steffel, B. 1984. *Handbook of gerontological nursing.* New York: Van Nostrand Reinhold.

Steffes, R. and Thralow, J. 1985. Do uniform colors keep patients awake? *Journal of Gerontological Nursing* 11(7):6-9.

Steinke, E.E. 1988. Older adults' knowledge and attitudes about sexuality and aging. *Image: The Journal of Nursing Scholarship* 20:93-95.

Stoneberg, C.; Pitcook, N.; and Myton, C. 1986. Pressure sores in the homebound: One solution. *American Journal of Nursing* 86(4):426-428.

Storm, D.; Metzger, B.; and Therrien, B. 1989. Effects of age on autonomic cardiovascular responsiveness in healthy men and women. *Nursing Research* 38(6):326-330.

Struble, L. and Sivertsen, L. 1987. Agitation behaviors in confused elderly patients. *Journal of Gerontological Nursing* 13(11):40-44.

Strumps, N.E. and Evans, L.K. 1988. Physical restraint of the hospitalized elderly: Perceptions of patients and nurses. *Nursing Research* 37(3):132-137.

Stull, M. and Vernon, J. 1986. Nursing care needs are changing in facilities with rising patient acuity. *Journal of Gerontological Nursing* 12(2):15-19.

Sullivan, J. and Armignacco, F. 1979. Effectiveness of a comprehensive health program for the well elderly by community health nurses. *Nursing Research* 28(2):70-75.

Terpstra, T.; Terpstra, T.; Plawecki, H.; and Streeter, J. 1989. As young as you feel: Age identification among the elderly. *Journal of Gerontological Nursing* 15(12):4-10.

Thatcher, R. 1983. 98.6°F: What is normal? *Journal of Gerontological Nursing* 9(1):22-27.

Thee, K.G. and Obrecht, W. 1984. Using a patient routing list to document pre-operative instruction. *Quality Review Bulletin* 10(5):149-150.

Thomas, B. 1988. Self-esteem and life satisfaction. *Journal of Gerontological Nursing* 14(12):25-30.

Thomas, P.D. and Hooper, E.M. 1983. Healthy elderly: Social bonds and locus of control. *Research in Nursing and Health* 6(1):11-16.

Thornbury, J. and Martin, A. 1983. Do nurses make a difference? *Journal of Gerontological Nursing* 9(8):440-445.

Tolbert, B.M. 1984. Reality orientation and remotivation in a long-term care facility. *Nursing and Health Care* 5(1):40-44.

Trice, L.R.B. 1986. Human spirit as a meaningful experience to the elderly: A phenomenological study. *Dissertation Abstracts* 47(2):576B.

Trippet, S.E. 1989. Being aware: The meaning of the relationship between social support and health among independent older women. *Dissertation Abstracts* 49(8):3111B.

Uman, G. and Hazard, M. 1981. Lifestyle change in elderly hypertensive persons: A multifaceted treatment program. *Journal of Aging and Health Promotion*:87-99.

U.S. Congress, Office of Technology Assessment. 1986. *Nurse practitioners, physician assistants, and certified nurse-midwives: A policy analysis.* Washington, D.C.: U.S. Government Printing Office.

U.S. Department of Health and Human Services. 1988. *Secretary's commission on nursing: Final report, vol. 1.* Washington, D.C.: the Department.

U.S. Department of Health, Education, and Welfare. 1980. *Quality assurance in nursing: A selected bibliography.* Washington, D.C.: the Department.

Valanis, B. and Yeaworth, R. 1982. Ratings of physical and mental health in the older bereaved. *Research in Nursing and Health* 5:137-146.

Valanis, B.; Yeaworth, R.; and Mullis, M. 1987. Alcohol use among bereaved and nonbereaved older persons. *Journal of Gerontological Nursing* 13(5):26-32.

VanOrt, S. and Woodtli A. 1989. Home health care providing a missing link. *Journal of Gerontological Nursing* 15(9):4-9.

Ventura, M.; Young, D.; Feldman, M.; Pastore, P.; Pidula, S.; and Yates, M. 1984. Effectiveness of health promotion interventions. *Nursing Research* 33(3):162-167.

————. 1985. Cost savings as an indicator of successful nursing intervention. *Nursing Research* 34:50-53.

Ventura, M.R.; Hageman, P.T.; Slakter, M.J.; and Fox, R.N. 1982. Correlations of two quality of nursing care measures. *Research in Nursing and Health* 5(1):32-43.

Vermeersch, P.E. 1987. Development of a scale to measure confusion in hospitalized adults. *Dissertation Abstracts* 48:3709B.

Voelkel, D. 1978. A study of reality orientation and resocialization groups with confused elderly. *Journal of Gerontological Nursing* 4(3):13-18.

Walker, L. 1984. The relationships between reminiscing, health state, physical functioning and depression in older adults. *Dissertation Abstracts* 45(5):1432B.

Walker, S.; Volken, K.; Schrist, K.; and Pender, N. 1988. Health-promoting life styles of older adults: Comparisons with young and middle-aged adults, correlates and patterns. *Advances in Nursing Science* 11(1):76-90.

Walshe, A. and Rosen, H. 1979. A study of patient falls from bed. *Journal of Nursing Administration* 9(5):31-35.

Warner, S.L. 1987. A comparative study of widows' and widowers' perceived social support during the first year of bereavement. *Archives of Psychiatric Nursing* 1(4):241-250.

Weinberg, A.; Engingro, P.; Miller, R.; Weinberg, L.; and Parker, C. 1989. Death in the nursing home: senescence infection and other causes. *Journal of Gerontological Nursing* 15(4):12-16.

Wells, T.J.; Brink, C.A.; and Diokno, A.C. 1987. Urinary incontinence in elderly women: Clinical findings. *Journal of the American Geriatrics Society* 35(10):933-939.

White, H.E.; Thurston, N.E.; Blackmore, K.A.; Green, S.E.; and Hannah, K.J. 1987. Body temperature in the elderly surgical patient. *Research in Nursing and Health* 10:317-321.

Whiteneck, M.R. 1988. Integrating ethics with quality assurance in long-term care. *Quality Review Bulletin* 14(5):138-143.

Whitman, S. and Kursh, E.D. 1987. Curbing incontinence. *Journal of Gerontological Nursing* 13(4):35-40.

Williams, M.; Campbell, E.; Raynor, W.; Mlynarczyk, S.; and Ward, S. 1985. Reducing acute confusional states in elderly patients with hip fractures. *Research in Nursing and Health* 8:329-337.

Williams, M.; Campbell, E.; Raynor, W.; Muscholt, M.; Mlynarczyk, S.; and Crane, L. 1985. Predictors of acute confusional states in hospitalized elderly patients. *Research in Nursing and Health* 8:31-40.

Williams, M.; Holloway, J.; Winn, M.; Wolanin, M.; Lawler, M.; Westwick, C.; and Chin, M. 1979. Nursing activities and acute confusional states in elderly hip-fractured patients. *Nursing Research* 28(1):25-35.

Williams, M.; Ward, S.; and Campbell, E. 1988. Confusion: Testing versus observation. *Journal of Gerontological Nursing* 14(1):25-30.

Wilson, H.S. 1989a. Family caregiving for a relative with Alzheimer's dementia: Coping with negative choices. *Nursing Research* 38:94-98.

————. 1989b. Family caregivers: The experience of Alzheimer's disease. *Applied Nursing Research* 2(1):40-45.

Wilson, R.; Patterson, M.; and Alford, D. 1989. Services for maintaining independence. *Journal of Gerontological Nursing* 15(6):31-37.

Wiltzius, F.; Gambert, S.; and Duthie, E. 1981. The importance of resident placement within a skilled nursing facility. *Journal of the American Geriatrics Society* 29(9):418-421.

Winger, J. and Schirm, V. 1989. Managing aggressive elderly in long-term care. *Journal of Gerontological Nursing* 15(2):28-33.

Wirtz, B.J. 1987. Effects of air and water mattresses on thermal regulation. *Journal of Gerontological Nursing* 13(5):13-17.

Wolanin, M.O. 1983. Clinical geriatric nursing research. In *Annual review of nursing research,* ed. H. Werley and J. Fitzpatrick, pp. 75-99. New York: Springer.

Wolock, I.; Schlesinger, E.; Dinerman, M.; and Seaton, R. 1987. The posthospital needs and care of patients: Implications for discharge planning. *Social Work in Health Care* 12(4):61.

Woolferk, C. 1989. What you can expect of nurses aides. *Geriatric Nursing* 10(4):178-180.

Worcester, M.H. and Quayhagen, M.P. 1983. Correlates of caregiving satisfaction: Prerequisites to elderly home care. *Research in Nursing Health* 6(2):61-67.

Wright, L.K. 1990. Mental health in older spouses: The dynamic interplay of resources, depression, quality of the marital relationship, and social participation. *Issues in Mental Health Nursing* 11(1):49-70.

Yauger, R.A. 1984. Non-nursing clerical functions: Time, cost, and effect on patient care. *Quality Review Bulletin* 10(2):54-56.

Young, S.; Muir-Nash, J.; and Ninos, M. 1988. Managing nocturnal wandering behavior. *Journal of Gerontological Nursing* 4(3):6-12.

Yu, L.C 1987. Incontinence stress index: Measuring psychological impact. *Journal of Gerontological Nursing* 13(7):18-25.

Yu, L.C. and Kaltreider, D.L. 1987. Stressed nurses: Dealing with incontinent patients. *Journal of Gerontological Nursing* 13(1):27-30.

Yu, L.C.; Kaltreider, D.L.; Lynne, D.; Hu, T.K.; Igou, J.F.; and Craighead, W.E. 1989. Measuring stress associated with incontinence. *Journal of Gerontological Nursing* 15(2):9-15.

Yurick, R.; Robs, S.; Spear, B.; and Ebert, N. 1980. *The aged person and the nursing process.* New York: Appleton Century Crofts.

Zepelin, H.; Wolfe, C.; and Kleinplatz, F. 1981. Evaluation of a year-long reality orientation program. *Journal of Gerontology* 36(1):70-77.

Zimmer, J.; Watson, N.; and Treat, A. 1984. Behavioral problems among patients in skilled nursing facilities. *American Journal of Public Health* 74(10):1118-1121.

Zimmerman, L.; Pozehl, B.; Duncan, K.; and Schmitz, R. 1989. Effects of music on patients who had chronic cancer pain. *Western Journal of Nursing Research* 11(3):298-309.

Zucker, J.S. 1987. The investigation of the relationships among social isolation and loneliness, acceptance of self and acceptance of others in the community elderly. *Dissertation Abstracts* 48(5):1305B.

Bibliography (by Quality of Care Research Areas)

Table 2.1 / Underuse: Home Health

Bredow, T.S. 1989. Prospective payment policy and the home health care of chronically ill patients. *Dissertation Abstracts* 49(8):3101B.

Card, D.A. 1987. Underutilization of health care services. *Dissertation Abstracts* 47(8):3292B.

Feldman, R.; Weiss, E.; and Small, N. 1989. Home care support program for frail elderly clients. *Applied Nursing Research* 2(1):48-49.

Gorenberg, B.D. 1986. Health maintenance of the frail elderly: Informal and formal help at home. *Dissertation Abstracts* 47(1):132-133B.

Moyer, N.C. 1987. Outcomes after termination of Medicare home health services: Their relationship to the resources and well-being of elderly caregiving spouses. *Dissertation Abstracts* 47:2840B.

Preston, D. and Grimes, J. 1987. A study in differences in social support. *Journal of Gerontological Nursing* 13(2):36-40.

VanOrt, S. and Woodtli A. 1989. Home health care—providing a missing link. *Journal of Gerontological Nursing* 15(9):4-9.

Wolock, I.; Schlesinger, E.; Dinerman, M.; and Seaton, R. 1987. The posthospital needs and care of patients: Implications for discharge planning. *Social Work in Health Care* 12(4):61.

Table 2.2 / Underuse: Elderly Women

Denny, M.; Koren, M.E.; and Wisby, M. 1989. Gynecological health needs of elderly women. *Journal of Gerontological Nursing* 15(1):33-38.

Packard, J. 1988. Health care system dependency among older adults: Patterns of hospital use by lung cancer patients. *Dissertation Abstracts* 48(2):363B.

Pasquale, D.K. 1987. A basis for prospective payment for home care. *Image: The Journal of Nursing Scholarship* 19:186-191.

Table 2.3 / Underuse: Diagnosis

Faherty, B.S. and Grier, M.G. 1984. Analgesic medication for elderly people postsurgery. *Nursing Research* 33(6):369-372.

Palmateer, L.M. and McCartney, J.R. 1985. Do nurses know when patients have cognitive deficits? *Journal of Gerontological Nursing* 11(2):6-16.

Reed, A.T. and Birge, S. 1988. Screening for osteoporosis. *Journal of Gerontological Nursing* 14(7):18-20.

Scura, K. and Wipple, B. 1990. Older adults as an HIV-positive risk group. *Journal of Gerontological Nursing* 16(2):6-10.

Table 3.1 / Overuse: Length of Stay

Edwardson, S.R. 1988. Outcomes of coronary care in the acute care setting. *Research in Nursing and Health* 11(4):215-222.

Grau, L. and Kobner, C. 1986. Comorbidity and length of stay: A case study. *Nursing and Health Care* 7(8):427-430.

Hobler, K.E. and Howlett, P.A. 1985. Surgery in the very elderly. *Quality Review Bulletin* 11(11):339-341.

Hogan, A.J. and Smith, D.W. 1987. Patient classification and resource allocation in Veterans Administration nursing homes. *Advances in Nursing Science* 9(3):56-71.

Lamont, C.T.; Sampson, S.; Matthias, R.; and Kane, R. 1983. The outcome of hospitalization for acute illness in the elderly. *Journal of the American Geriatric Society* 31:282-288.

Leslie, F. 1981. Nursing diagnosis: Use in long-term care. *American Journal of Nursing* 81(5):1012-1014.

Marchette, L. and Holloman, F. 1986. Length of stay: Significant variables. *Journal of Nursing Administration* 16(3):12-20.

Micheletti, J.A. and Shlala, T.J. 1986. RUGS II: Implications for management and quality in long term care. *Quality Review Bulletin* 12(7):235-242.

Neildinger, S.H.; Scroggins, K.; and Kennedy, L.M. 1987. Cost evaluation of discharge planning for hospitalized elderly. *Nursing Economic$* 5:225-230.

Nosek, L.J. 1987. Explanation of hospital stay by nursing diagnoses, medical diagnoses, and social position. *Dissertation Abstracts* 47(7):2840B.

Ventura, M.R.; Young, D.E.; Feldman, M.J.; Pastore, P.; Pidula, S.; and Yates, M.A.1985. Cost savings as an indicator of successful nursing intervention. *Nursing Research* 34:50-53.

Table 3.2 / Overuse: Hospitalization and Costs

Brands, R. 1983. Acceptance of nurses as primary-care providers by retired people. *Advances in Nursing Science* 5(3):37-49.

Cleveland, S.A. 1988. Assessment of self-care agency in patients with chronic obstructive pulmonary disease. *Dissertation Abstracts* 49(6):2124B.

Collard, A.F. 1989. Predicting readmissions of elderly patients to the acute care hospital. *Dissertation Abstracts* 49(8):3101B.

Collard, A.F.; Bachman, S.S.; and Beatrice, D.F. 1985. Acute care delivery for the geriatric patient: An innovative approach. *Quality Review Bulletin* 11(6):180-185.

Igou, J.; Hawkins, J.; Johnson, E.; and Utley, Q. 1989. Nurse-managed approach to care. *Geriatric Nursing* 10(1):32-34.

Kline, N.W. 1989. Psychophysiological processes of stress in people with a chronic physical illness. *Dissertation Abstracts* 49(6):2129B.

Schwartz, R.; Zaremba, M.; and Ra, K. 1985. Third-party coverage for diabetes education programs. *Quality Review Bulletin* 11(7):213-216.

Thornbury, J. and Martin, A. 1983. Do nurses make a difference? *Journal of Gerontological Nursing* 9(8):440-445.

Ventura, M.R.; Young, D.E.; Feldman, M.J.; Pastore, P.; Pidula, S.; and Yates, M.A.1985. Cost savings as an indicator of successful nursing intervention.*Nursing Research* 34:50-53.

Table 3.3 / Overuse: Restraint and Medication Usage

Brown, M. and Everett I. 1990. Gentler bowel fitness with fiber. *Geriatric Nursing* 11(1):26-27.

Butler, F.; Burgio, L.; and Engel, B. 1987. Neuroleptics and behavior: A comparative study.*Journal of Gerontological Nursing* 13(6):15-19.

Chisholm, M.; Lundin, S.; and Wood, J. 1983. Withdrawing digoxin: Worth a try. *Geriatric Nursing* 4(5):290-292.

Clapin-French, E. 1986. Sleep patterns of aged persons in long-term care facilities.*Journal of Advanced Nursing* 11:57-66.

Keenan, R.; Redshaw, A.; Munson, J.; and Mundt, W. 1983. The benefits of a drug holiday. *Geriatric Nursing* 4(2):103-104.

Strumps, N.E. and Evans, L.K. 1988. Physical restraint of the hospitalized elderly: Perceptions of patients and nurses.*Nursing Research* 37(3):132-137.

Table 3.4 / Overuse: DRG-Related Studies

Fitzgerald, J.; Moore, P.; and Dittus, R. 1988. The care of elderly patients with hip fractures: Changes since implementation of the prospective payment system. *New England Journal of Medicine* November:1392-1397.

Gamroth, S.L. 1988. Long-term care resource requirements before and after the prospective payment system.*Image: The Journal of Nursing Scholarship* 20(1):7-11.

Harron, J. and Schaeffer, J. 1986. DRGs in the intensity of skilled nursing. *Geriatric Nursing* 7(1):31-33.

McGovern, K. and Newbern, V. 1988. Long-term care facility: DRG impact.*Journal of Gerontological Nursing* 14(9):17-20.

Stull, M. and Vernon, J. 1986. Nursing care needs are changing in facilities with rising patient acuity. *Journal of Gerontological Nursing* 12(2):15-19.

Weinberg, A.; Engingro, P.; Miller, R.; Weinberg, L.; and Parker,C. 1989. Death in the nursing home: senescence, infection, and other causes. *Journal of Gerontological Nursing* 15(4):12-16.

Table 4.1 / Technical Quality of Care: Quality of Life, Life Satisfaction, and Health Promotion

Bowsher, J. 1987. Personal control and psychological well-being of institutionalized elders. *Dissertation Abstracts* 48(5):1299B.

Brown, M. and Everett I. 1990. Gentler bowel fitness with fiber. *Geriatric Nursing* 11(1):26-27.

Cassels, H.B. 1988. Health beliefs and osteoporosis prevention by menopausal women. *Dissertation Abstracts* 49(6):2123.

Chang, B.L. 1978. Generalized expectancy, situational perception, and morale among institutionalized elderly. *Nursing Research* 27(5):316-324.

Chang, B.L.; Uman, G.C.; Linn, L.S.; Ware, J.E.; and Kane, R.L. 1985. Adherence to health care regimens among elderly women. *Nursing Research* 34(1):27-31.

Dean, H. 1988. Multiple instruments for measuring quality of life. In *Instruments for clinical nursing,* ed. M. Frank-Stromborg, pp. 97-105. Norwalk, Conn.: Appleton & Lange.

Devey, S. 1990. Older lesbian women: An invisible minority. *Journal of Gerontological Nursing* 16(5):35-39.

Dolinsky, E. 1987. The relationships of perceived social support and self-disclosure to the morale of older women. *Dissertation Abstracts* 48(3):702B.

Ferrans, C.E.; Powers, M.J.; and Kasch, C.R. 1987. Satisfaction with health care of hemodialysis patients. *Research in Nursing and Health* 10(6):367-374.

Flynn, M.K. and Frantz, R. 1987. Coronary artery bypass surgery: Quality of life during early convalescence. *Heart and Lung* 16:159-167.

Flynn, R. 1986. The relationship of self-actualization, internal locus of control, and sexual activity to the experience of life satisfaction in elderly men. *Dissertation Abstracts*

Folden, S. 1990. On the inside looking out: Perceptions of the home bound. *Journal of Gerontological Nursing* 16(1):15-19.

Forsyth, G.L.; Delaney, K.D.; and Gresham, M.L. 1984. Vying for a winning position: Management style of the chronically ill. *Research in Nursing and Health* 7(3):181-188.

Foster, M.F. 1987. The study of relationships among perceived current health, health promoting activities, and life satisfaction in older black adults. *Dissertation Abstracts* 48(5):1301B.

Frank-Stromborg, M. 1988. Single instruments for measuring quality of life. In *Instruments for clinical nursing research,* ed. M. Frank-Stromborg, pp. 779-795. Norwalk, Conn.: Appleton & Lange.

Fuller, S.S. and Larson, S.B. 1980. Life events, emotional support, and health of older people. *Research in Nursing and Health* 3(2):81-89.

Gilson, P. and Coats, S. 1980. A study of morale in low income blacks. *Journal of Gerontological Nursing* 6(7):385-388.

Hargrove-Huttle, R. 1989. Virginia Henderson's nature of nursing theory and quality of life for the older adult. *Dissertation Abstracts* 49(8):3104B.

Hoeffer, B. 1987. Predictors of life outlook of older single women. *Research in Nursing and Health* 10(2):111-117.

Horgan, P. 1987. Health status perceptions affect health-related behaviors. *Journal of Gerontological Nursing* 13(12):30-33.

Johnson, B.K. 1987. The sexual interest, participation, and satisfaction of older men and women. *Dissertation Abstracts* 47(12):4824B.

Johnson, F.; Cloyd, C.; and Wer, J. 1982. Life satisfaction of poor urban black aged. *Advances in Nursing Science* 4(3):27-35.

Johnson, F.L.; Foxall, M.J.; Kidwell-Udin, M.A.; Miller, G.; and Stolzer, M.E. 1984. Life satisfaction in the minority elderly. *Issues in Mental Health Nursing* 6(1-2):189-207.

Keller, M.; Levinthal, H.; Prohaska, T.; and Linthal, E. 1989. Beliefs about aging and illness in a community sample. *Research in Nursing and Health* 12(4):247-255.

King, F.E.; Figge, J.; and Harman, P. 1986. The elderly coping at home: A study of continuity of nursing care. *Journal of Advanced Nursing* 11:41-46.

Laborde, J.M. and Powers, M. J. 1985. Life satisfaction, health control orientation, and illness-related factors in persons with osteoarthritis. *Research in Nursing and Health* 8(2):183-190.

Lacey, A.L. 1989. Health beliefs and health behavior in elderly, chronically ill males. *Dissertation Abstracts* 49(8):3106B.

Magilvy, J. 1985. Quality of life of hearing-impaired older women. *Nursing Research* 34(3):140-144.

McDaniel, R.W. 1987. Relationship of participation in health promotion behaviors to quality of life. *Dissertation Abstracts* 48(7):1040B.

Mills, R. 1986. The relationship of interpersonal time, life position, and stroking to life satisfaction of older individuals. *Dissertation Abstracts* 46:2625B.

O'Connell, K.; Hamera, E.; Kanapp, T.; Cassmeyer, V.; Eaks, G.; and Fox, M. 1984. Symptom use and self-regulation in Type 2 diabetes. *Advances in Nursing Science* 3(3):19-28.

Oudt, B.M. 1989. Self-reported health status and health behaviors of women aged 85 years and older. *Dissertation Abstracts* 49(7):2569B.

Padilla, G.V. and Grant, M.M. 1985. Quality of life as a cancer nursing outcome variable. *Advances in Nursing Science* 8(1):15-24.

Pascucci, M.A. 1988. Health values, incentives, and social support related to health promotions behaviors in the well elderly. *Dissertation Abstracts* 46(4):1006B.

Pohl, J.M. and Fuller, S.S. 1980. Perceived choice, social interaction, and dimensions of morale of residents in a home for the aged. *Research in Nursing and Health* 3(4):147-157.

Rauckhorst, L. 1987. Health habits of elderly widows. *Journal of Gerontological Nursing* 13(8):19-22.

Ryden, M. 1984. Morale and perceived control in institutionalized elderly. *Nursing Research* 33(3):130-136.

Ryden, M.B. 1985. Environmental support for autonomy in the institutionalized elderly. *Research in Nursing and Health* 8:363-371.

Schafer, S. 1989. An aggressive approach to promoting health responsibility. *Journal of Gerontological Nursing* 15(4):22-27.

Schank, M. and Lough, M. 1989. Maintaining health and independence of elderly women. *Journal of Gerontological Nursing* 15(6):8-11.

Schwartz, D. 1980. Hamlet dweller-city dweller. *Geriatric Nursing* 1(2):128-132.

Schwirian, P. 1982. Life satisfaction among nursing home residents. *Geriatric Nursing* 3(2):111-117.

Sellers, J.B. 1986. The influence of a confidante on the morale of institutionalized elderly women. *Dissertation Abstracts* 47(4):1492B.

Simon, J. 1990. Humor and its relationship to perceived health, life satisfaction, and morale in older adults. *Issues in Mental Health Nursing* 11(1):17-31.

Speake, D.; Cowart, M.; and Pellet, K. 1989. Health perceptions and life styles of the elderly. *Research in Nursing and Health* 12(2):93-100.

Spitzer, W.; Dobston, A.; Hall, J.; Chesterman, E.; Levi, J.; and Shepherd, R. 1981. Measuring the quality of life of cancer patients: A concise QL-index for use byphysicians. *Journal of Chronic Disease* 34(12):585-597.

Steinke, E. E. 1988. Older adults' knowledge and attitudes about sexuality and aging. *Image: The Journal of Nursing Scholarship* 20:93-95.

Terpstra, T.; Terpstra, T.; Plawecki, H.; and Streeter, J. 1989. As young as you feel: Age identification among the elderly. *Journal of Gerontological Nursing* 15(12):4-10.

Thomas, B. 1988. Self-esteem and life satisfaction. *Journal of Gerontological Nursing* 14(12):25-30.

Thomas, P.D. and Hooper, E.M. 1983. Healthy elderly: Social bonds and locus of control. *Research in Nursing and Health* 6(1):11-16.

Trice, L.R.B. 1986. Human spirit as a meaningful experience to the elderly: A phenomenological study. *Dissertation Abstracts* 47(2):576B.

Trippet, S.E. 1989. Being aware: The meaning of the relationship between social support and health among independent older women. *Dissertation Abstracts* 49(8):3111B.

Walker, S.; Volken, K.; Schrist, K.; and Pender, N. 1988. Health-promoting life styles of older adults: Comparisons with young and middle-aged adults, correlates, and patterns. *Advances in Nursing Science* 11(1):76-90.

Table 4.2. / Technical Quality of Care: Mental Health of Older People

Braun, J.V. 1987. Failure to thrive aged in nursing home. *Dissertation Abstracts* 48(1):143B.

Burckhardt, C.S. 1987. The effect of therapy on the mental health of the elderly. *Research in Nursing and Health* 10(4):277-285.

Cassels, C.; Fortinash, K.; and Eckstein, A. 1981. Retirement: Aspects, responses, and nursing implications. *Journal of Gerontological Nursing* 7(6):355.

Christian, E.; Dluhy, N.; and O'Neill, R. 1989. Sounds of silence: Coping with hearing loss and loneliness. *Journal of Gerontological Nursing* 15(11):4-9.

Christman, N.J.; McConnell, E.A.; Pfeiffer, C.; Webster, K.K.; Schmitt, M.; and Ries,J. 1988. Uncertainty, coping, and distress following myocardial infarction: Transition from hospital to home. *Research in Nursing & Health* 11:71-82.

Collins, M. 1988. Humor: An informal channel of communication used by institutionalized aged to express feelings of aggression due to personal deficits in power and states. *Dissertation Abstracts* 49(5):1619B.

Daily, E. and Futrell, M. 1989. Retirement attitudes and health status of pre-retired and retired men and women. *Journal of Gerontological Nursing* 15(1):29-32.

Dietx, M. 1986. Sources of stress among older rural women in North Dakota. *Dissertation Abstracts* 47(4):1486B.

Farran, C. and McCann, J. 1989. Longitudinal analysis of hope in community-based older adults. *Archives of Psychiatric Nursing* 3(5):272-276.

Farran, C. and Popovich, J. 1990. Hope: A relevant concept for geriatric psychiatry. *Archives of Psychiatric Nursing* 4(2):124-130.

Farran, C.; Salloway, J.; and Clark, D. 1990. Measurement of hope in a community-based older population. *Western Journal of Nursing Research* 12(1):42-59.

Fishman, S. 1989. An investigation of the relationships among an older adult's lifereview, ego integrity, and death anxiety. *Dissertation Abstracts* 49(8):3103B.

Greene, V. and Monahan, D. 1982. The impact of visitation on patient well-being in nursing homes. *The Gerontologist* 22(4):418-423.

Hoeffer, B. 1987. Predictors of life outlook of older single women. *Research in Nursing and Health* 10(2):111-117.

Keane, S. and Sells, S. 1990. Recognizing depression in the elderly. *Journal of Gerontological Nursing* 16(1):21-25.

Leja, A. 1989. Using guided imagery to combat postsurgical depression. *Journal of Gerontological Nursing* 15(4):6-11.

Louis, M. 1981. Personal space boundary needs of elderly persons: An empirical study. *Journal of Gerontological Nursing* 7(7):395-400.

Nelson, P. 1989. Ethnic differences in intrinsic/extrinsic religious orientation and depression in the elderly. *Archives of Psychiatric Nursing* 3(4):199-204.

———.1990. Intrinsic/extrinsic religious orientation of the elderly: Relationship to depression and self-esteem. *Journal of Gerontological Nursing* 16(2):29-35.

Newman, M.A. and Gaudiano, J.K. 1984. Depression as an explanation for decreased subjective time in the elderly. *Nursing Research* 33(3):137-139.

Powers, B.A. 1988. Social network, social support, in elderly institutionalized people. *Advances in Nursing Science* 10(2):40-58.

Poznanski, C. 1987. Types and meanings of caring behaviors among elderly nursing home residents. *Dissertation Abstracts* 48(6):1643B.

Preston, D. and Dellasega, C. 1990. Elderly women in stress: Does marriage make a difference? *Journal of Gerontological Nursing* 16(4):26-32.

Rainwater, A.J. 1988. Elderly loneliness and its relation to residential care. *Journal of Gerontological Nursing* 6(10):593-599.

Reed, P. 1989. Mental health of older adults. *Western Journal of Nursing Research* 11(2):143-163.

Reed, P.G. 1986a. Developmental resources and depression in the elderly. *Nursing Research* 35(6):368-374.

———.1986b. Religiousness among terminally ill and healthy adults. *Research in Nursing and Health* 9(1):9, 35-41.

Rodgers, B. 1989. Loneliness: Easing the pain of the hospitalized elderly. *Journal of Gerontological Nursing* 15(8):16-21.

Scott, D.W.; Oberst, M.T.; and Bookbinder, M.I. 1984. Stress-coping response to genitourinary carcinoma in men. *Nursing Research* 33(6):325-329.

Slimmer, L.; Edwards-Beckett, J.; LeSage, J.; Ellor, J.; and Lopez, M. 1990. Helping those who don't help themselves. *Geriatric Nursing* 11(1):20-22.

Slimmer, L.; Lopez, M.; LeSage, J.; and Ellor, J. 1987. Perceptions of learned helplessness. *Journal of Gerontological Nursing* 13(5):33-37.

Wright, L.K. 1990. Mental health in older spouses: The dynamic interplay of resources, depression, quality of the marital relationship, and social participation. *Issues in Mental Health Nursing* 11(1):49-70.

Zucker, J.S. 1987. The investigation of the relationships among social isolation and loneliness, acceptance of self and acceptance of others in the community elderly. *Dissertation Abstracts* 48(5):1305B.

Table 4.3 / Technical Quality of Care: Relaxation and Multimethod Nursing

DeMoss, C.J. 1980. Giving intravenous chemotherapy at home. *American Journal of Nursing* 80(12):2188-2189.

Dixon, J. 1984. Effect of nursing interventions on nutritional and performance status in cancer patients. *Nursing Research* 33:330-335.

Fakouri, C. and Jones, P. 1987. Relaxation treatment: Slow stroke back rub. *Journal of Gerontological Nursing* 13(2):32-35.

Frank, J. 1985. The effects of music therapy and guided visual imagery on chemotherapy-induced nausea and vomiting. *Oncology Nursing Forum* 12(5):47-52.

Hamilton, J. 1989. Comfort and the hospitalized chronically ill. *Journal of Gerontological Nursing* 15(4):28-33.

Kutlenios, R.M. 1985. A comparison of holistic, mental, and physical health nursing interventions with the elderly. *Dissertation Abstracts* 46:995B.

Rice, V.H.; Caldwell, M.; Butler, S.; and Robinson, J. 1986. Relaxation training and response to cardiac catheterization: A pilot study. *Nursing Research* 35(1):39-43.

Zimmerman, L.; Pozehl, B.; Duncan, K.; and Schmitz, R. 1989. Effects of music on patients who had chronic cancer pain. *Western Journal of Nursing Research* 11(3):298-309.

Table 4.4 / Technical Quality of Care: Self-Care and Activities of Daily Living

Buckwalter, K.; Cusack, D.; Stidles, E.; Wadle, K.; and Beaver, M. 1989. Increasing communication ability in aphasic/dysarthric patients. *Western Journal of Nursing Research* 11(6):736-747.

Colling, J.C. 1985. Elderly nursing home residents' control of activities of daily living and well-being. *Dissertation Abstracts* 46(10):3389-3390B.

Davidson, A.W. and Young, C. 1985. Repatterning of stroke rehabilitation clients following return to life in the community. *Journal of Neurosurgical Nursing* 17:123-128.

DeVon, H.A. and Powers, M.J. 1984. Health beliefs, adjustment to illness, and control of hypertension. *Research in Nursing and Health* 7(1):10-16.

Hain, M.J. and Chen, S.C. 1986. Health needs of the elderly. *Nursing Research* 25(6):433-439.

Harrell, J.; McConnell, E.; Wildman, D.; and Samsa, G. 1989. Do nursing diagnoses affect functional status? *Journal of Gerontological Nursing* 15(10):13-19.

Hess, P. 1986. Chinese and Hispanic elders and OTC drugs. *Geriatric Nursing* 7(6):314-318.

Johnson, J. and Moore, J. 1988. The drug taking practices in the rural elderly. *Applied Nursing Research* 1(3):128-131.

Karl, C. 1982. The effect of an exercise program on self-care activities for the institutionalized elderly. *Journal of Gerontological Nursing* 8(5):282-285.

Kelly-Hayes, M. 1987. Quality of survivorship following stroke: Cognitive, physical, and social factors. *Dissertation Abstracts* 48(4):1004B.

King, K.B.; Norsen, L.H.; Robertson, R.K.; and Hicks, G.L. 1987. Patient management of pain medication after cardiac surgery. *Nursing Research* 36(3):145-150.

Labi, M.; Phillips, T.; and Gresham, G. 1980. Psychosocial disability in physically restored long-term stroke survivors. *Archives of Physical Medicine Rehabilitation* 61:561-565.

Lambert, V.A. 1985. Study of factors associated with psychological well-being in rheumatoid arthritic women. *Image: The Journal of Nursing Scholarship* 17:50-53.

Lantz, J. 1985. In search of agents for self-care. *Journal of Gerontological Nursing* 11(7):10-13.

Lewis, M.A.; Kane, R.L.; Kretin, S.; and Clark, V. 1985. The immediate and subsequent outcomes of nursing home care. *American Journal of Public Health* 75(7):758-762.

Magilvy, J.; Brown, N.; and Dydyn, J. 1988. The experience of home health care: Perceptions of older adults. *Public Health Nursing* 5(3):140-145.

Mahoney, E.K. 1985. The interaction of physical illness, coping focus, and perceived social support and their relationship to recovery from stroke. *Dissertation Abstracts* 47(5):1929B.

Mion, L.; Frengley, J.D.; and Adams, M. 1986. Nursing patients 75 years and older. *Nursing Management* 17(9):24-28.

Patsdaughter, C. and Pesznecker, B. 1988. Medication regimes in the elderly homecare client. *Journal of Gerontological Nursing* 14(10):30-34.

Pensiero, M. and Adams, M. 1987. Dress and self-esteem. *Journal of Gerontological Nursing* 13(10):11-17.

Shamanasky, S. and Hamilton, W. 1979. The health behavioral awareness test: Self-care education for the elderly. *Journal of Gerontological Nursing* 5(1):29-32.

Table 4.5 / Technical Quality of Care: Food and Fluid Intake, Oral Hygiene

Adams, F. 1988. Fluid intake: How much do elders drink? *Geriatric Nursing* 9(4):218-221.

Athlin, E.; Norberg, A.; Axelsson, K.; Moller, A.; and Nordstrom, G. 1989. Aberrant eating behavior in elderly Parkinsonian patients with and without dementia: Analysis of video-recorded meals. *Research in Nursing and Health* 12(1):12,41-51.

Brown, C.S.B. and Stegman, M.R. 1988. Nutritional assessment of surgical patients. *Quality Review Bulletin* 14(10):302-306.

Cagawa-Busby, K.; Heltkempr, M.; Hansen, B.; Hanson, R.; and Vanderburg, V. 1988. Effects of diet temperature on tolerance of enteral feedings. *Nursing Research* 29(5):276-280.

Collinsworth, R. and Boyle, K. 1989. Nutritional assessment of the elderly. *Journal of Gerontological Nursing* 15(12):17-21.

DeWalt, E. 1975. Effect of timed hygiene measures on oral mucosa in a group of elderly subjects. *Nursing Research* 24:104-108.

Eaton, M.; Mitchell-Bonair, I.L.; and Friedmann, E. 1986. The effect of touch on nutritional intake of chronic organic brain syndrome patients. *Journal of Gerontology* 41(5):611.

Flynn, K.T.; Norton, L.C.; and Fisher, R.L. 1987. Enternal tube feeding: Indications, practices, and outcomes. *Image: The Journal of Nursing Scholarship* 19:16-19.

Gasper, P.M. 1988. Fluid intake: What determines how much patients drink? *Geriatric Nursing* 9(4):221-224.

Howe, M.; Coulton, M.; Almon, G.; and Sandrick, K.M. 1980b. Use of scaled out come criteria for a target patient population. *Quality Review Bulletin* 6(4):15-21.

Longman, A. and DeWalt, E. 1986. A guide for oral assessment. *Geriatric Nursing* 7(5):252-253.

Meyer, P.A. 1987. Nursing home residents' water intake. *Dissertation Abstracts* 47(3):996B.

Michaelsson, E.; Norberg, A.; and Norberg, B. 1987. Feeding methods for demented patients in end stage of life. *Geriatric Nursing* 8(2):69-73.

Pritchard, V. 1988. Tube feeding related pneumonias. *Journal of Gerontological Nursing* 14(7):32-36.

Spitzer, M.E. 1988. Taste acuity in institutionalized and noninstitutionalized elderly men. *Journal of Gerontology* 43(3):71-74.

Table 4.6 / Technical Quality of Care: Nocturnal Behavior

Clapin-French, E. 1986. Sleep patterns of aged persons in long-term care facilities. *Journal of Advanced Nursing* 11:57-66.

Gress, L.; Hassanein, R.; and Bahr, S.R. 1981. Nocturnal behavior of selected institutionalized adults. *Journal of Gerontological Nursing* 7(2):86-92.

Hayter, J. 1983. Sleep behaviors of older persons. *Nursing Research* 32(4):242-246.

Pacini, C. and Fitzpatrick, J. 1982. Sleep patterns of hospitalized and nonhospitalized aged individuals. *Journal of Gerontological Nursing* 8(6):327-332.

Young, S.; Muir-Nash, J.; and Ninos, M. 1988. Managing nocturnal wandering behavior. *Journal of Gerontological Nursing* 4(3):6-12.

Table 4.7 / Technical Quality of Care: Incontinence

Baigis-Smith, J.; Jakobac-Smith, D.; Rose, M.; and Newman, D. 1989. Managing urinary incontinence in community-residing elderly persons. *The Gerontologist* 29(2):229-233.

Barker, J. and Mitteness, L. 1989. Shedding light on nocturia. *Geriatric Nursing* 10(5):239-240.

Brink, C.; Sampselle, C.; Wells, T.; Diokno, A.; and Gillis, G. 1989. A digital test for pelvic muscle strength in older women with urinary incontinence. *Nursing Research* 38(4):196-199.

Burgio, L.; Jones, L.; and Engel, B. 1988. Studying incontinence in an urban nursing home. *Journal of Gerontological Nursing* 14(4):40-45.

Diokno, A.C.; Wells, T.J.; and Brink, C.A. 1987. Urinary incontinence in elderly women: Urodynamic evaluation. *Journal of the American Geriatrics Society* 35:940-946.

Grant, R. 1982. Washable pads or disposable diapers? *Geriatric Nursing* 3(4):248.

Gross, J. 1990. Bladder dysfunction after a stroke: It's not always inevitable. *Journal of Gerontological Nursing* 16(4):20-25.

Haeker, S. 1985. Disposable versus reusable incontinence products. *Geriatric Nursing* 6(6):345-347.

Hu, T.; Kaltreider, D.; and Igou, J. 1989. Incontinence products: Which is best? *Geriatric Nursing* 10(4):184-186.

————.1990. The cost-effectiveness of disposable versus reusable diapers: A controlled experiment in a nursing home. *Journal of Gerontological Nursing* 16(2):19-24.

Kaltreider, D.; Hu, T.; Igou, J.; Yu, L.; and Craighead, W. 1990. Can reminders curb incontinence? *Geriatric Nursing* 11(1):17-19.

Lara, L.; Troop, P.; and Beadleson-Baird, M. 1990. Risk of urinary tract infection in bowel incontinent men. *Journal of Gerontological Nursing* 16(5):14-26.

LeSage, J.; Slimmer, L.; Lopez, M.; and Ellor, J. 1989. Learned helplessness. *Journal of Gerontological Nursing* 15(5):16-23.

Long, M.L. 1985. Incontinence. *Journal of Gerontological Nursing* 11(1):30-41.

Miller, J. 1990. Assessing urinary incontinence. *Journal of Gerontological Nursing* 16(3):15-19.

Oberst, M.T.; Graham, D.; Geller, N.L.; Maus, W.; Stearns, M.W., Jr.; and Tiernan,E. 1981. Catheter management programs and postoperative urinary dysfunction. *Research in Nursing and Healthy* 4(1):175-181.

Ouslander, J.G.; Morishita, L.; Blaustein, J.; Orzeck, S.; Dunn, S.; and Sayre, J. 1987.Clinical, functional, and psychosocial characteristics of an incontinent nursing home population. *Journal of Gerontology* 42(6):631-637.

Pearson, B.D. and Droessler, D. 1988. Continence through nursing care. *Geriatric Nursing* 9(6):347-349.

Pritchard, V. 1985. Watch out! Urinary tract infections must not spread. *Journal of Gerontological Nursing* 11(5):16-19.

Robb, S.S. 1985. Urinary incontinence verification in elderly men. *Nursing Research* 34(5):278-282.

Schneille, J.; Traughper, B.; Morgan, D.; Embry, J.; Binion, A.; and Coleman, A.1983. Management of geriatric incontinence in nursing homes. *Journal of Applied Behavioral Analysis* 16(2):235-241.

Simons, J. 1985. Does incontinence affect your client's self-concept? *Journal of Gerontological Nursing* 11(6):37-40.

Sowell, V.A.; Schnelle, J.F.; Hu, T.; and Traughber, B. 1987. A cost comparison of five methods of managing urinary incontinence. *Quality Review Bulletin* 13(12):411-414.

Wells, T.J.; Brink, C.A.; and Diokno, A.C. 1987. Urinary incontinence in elderly women: Clinical findings. *Journal of the American Geriatrics Society* 35(10):933-939.

Whitman, S. and Kursh, E.D. 1987. Curbing incontinence. *Journal of Gerontological Nursing* 13(4):35-40.

Yu, L.C. 1987. Incontinence stress index: Measuring psychological impact. *Journal of Gerontological Nursing* 13(7):18-25.

Yu, L.C. and Kaltreider, D.L. 1987. Stressed nurses: Dealing with incontinent patients. *Journal of Gerontological Nursing* 13(1):27-30.

Yu, L.C.; Kaltreider, D.L.; Lynne, D.; Hu, T.K.; Igou, J.F.; and Craighead, W.E. 1989. Measuring stress associated with incontinence. *Journal of Gerontological Nursing* 15(2):9-15.

Table 4.8 / Technical Quality of Care: Pressure Sores

Allman, R.; Walker, J.; Hart, M.; Laprade, C.; Knoll, L.; and Smith, C. 1987. Air fluidized beds or conventional therapy for pressure sores: A randomized trial. *Annals of Internal Medicine* 107:641-648.

Becker, L. and Goodemote, C. 1984. Treating pressure sores with or without antacid. *American Journal of Nursing* 84(3):351-352.

Bergstrom, N.; Braden, B.; Laguzza, A.; and Holman, V. 1987. The Braden scale for predicting pressure sore risk. *Nursing Research* 36(4):205-210.

Black, M.; VanBerkel, C.; Green, E.; Everett, I.; and Krilyk J. 1987. Criteria map—potential for skin breakdown: A quality assurance tool for use in any setting. *Quality Review Bulletin* 15(11):340-345.

Blom, M.F. 1985. Dramatic decrease in decubitus ulcers. *Geriatric Nursing* 6(2):84-87.

Bristow, J.; Goldfarb, E.; and Green, M. 1987. Clinitron therapy: Is it effective? *Geriatric Nursing* 8(3):120-124.

Brown, M.; Boosinger, J.; Black, J.; and Gaspar, T. 1985. Nursing innovation for prevention of decubitus ulcers in long-term care facilities. *Plastic Surgical Nursing* Summer:57-64.

Clarke, M. 1988. The nursing prevention of pressure sores in hospital and community patients. *Journal of Advanced Nursing* 13:365-373.

Diekmann, J.M. 1984. Use of a dental irrigating device in the treatment of decubitus ulcers. *Nursing Research* 33(5):303-305.

Distel, L. 1982. A nursing quality assurance investigation of orthopedic patient care. *Quality Review Bulletin* 8(10):20-22.

Droessler, D. and Maibusch, R.M. 1982. Development of a nursing care plan for healing and preventing decubiti. *Quality Review Bulletin Special Edition* Spring:21-25.

Frantz, R.A. and Kinney, C.K. 1986. Variables associated with skin dryness in the elderly. *Nursing Research* 35(2):98-100.

Hyland, D. and Kirkland, V.J. 1980. Infrared therapy for skin ulcers. *American Journal of Nursing*

Munro, B.; Brown, L.; and Heitman, B. 1989. Pressure ulcers: one bed or another? *Geriatric Nursing* 10(4):190-192.

Pajk, M.; Craven, G.A.; Cameron, J.; Shipps, T.; and Bennum, N.W. 1986. Investigating the problem of pressure sores. *Journal of Gerontological Nursing* 12(7):11-16.

Reynolds, M. 1989. Eliminating pressure sore risk. In *Research review: Studies for nursing practice,* ed. L. Cronenwett, p. 3. Baltimore: Williams & Wilkins.

Stoneberg, C.; Pitcook, N.; and Myton, C. 1986. Pressure sores in the homebound: One solution. *American Journal of Nursing* 86(4):426-428.

Wirtz, B.J. 1987. Effects of air and water mattresses on thermal regulation. *Journal of Gerontological Nursing* 13(5):13-17.

Table 4.9 / Technical Quality of Care: Thermoregulation and Cardiovascular Parameters

Banasik, J. and Steadman, R. 1987. Effect of position on arterial oxygenation in postoperative coronary revascularization patients. *Heart and Lung* 16(6):652-657.

Biddle, C. and Biddle, W. 1985. A plastic head cover to reduce surgical heat loss. *Geriatric Nursing* 6(1):39-41.

Davis, C. and Lentz, M. 1989. Circadian rhythms: charting oral temperatures to spot abnormalities. *Journal of Gerontological Nursing* 15(4):34-39.

Doering, L. and Dracup, K. 1988. Comparisons of cardiac output in supine and lateral positions. *Nursing Research* 37(2):114-118.

Dressler, D.K.; Smejkal, C.; and Ruffolo, M.L. 1983. A comparison of oral and rectal temperature measurement on patients receiving oxygen by mask. *Nursing Research* 32(6):373 375.

Durham, M.L.; Swanson, B.; and Pulford, N. 1986. Effects of tachypnea on oral temperature estimation: A replication. *Nursing Research* 35(4):211-214.

Folta, A.; Metzger, B.; and Therrien, B. 1989. Pre-existing physical activity level and cardiovascular responses across the Valsalva maneuver. *Nursing Research* 38(3):139-143.

Folta, A.; Storm, D.; and Therrien, B. 1987. The effect of aging on the intensity of cardiovascular responses during the Valsalva maneuver in healthy adults. *Heart and Lung* 16(3): 330-331.

Heidenreich, T. and Giuffre, M. 1990. Postoperative temperature measurement. *Nursing Research* 39(3):153-155.

Higgins, P. 1983. Can 98.6oF be a fever in disguise? *Geriatric Nursing* 4(2):101-102.

Polyneaux, R.; Papciak, B.; and Woem, D. 1987. Coagulation studies and the in dwelling heparinized catheter. *Heart and Lung* 16(1):20-23.

Schneider, J. 1987. Effects of caffeine ingestion on heart rate, blood pressure, mildcardio-oxygen consumption, and cardiac rhythm in acute mild cardio-infarction patients. *Heart and Lung* 16(2):167-174.

Storm, D.; Metzger, B.; and Therrien, B. 1989. Effects of age on autonomic cardiovascular responsiveness in healthy men and women. *Nursing Research* 38(6):326-330.

Thatcher, R. 1983. 98.6oF: What is normal? *Journal of Gerontological Nursing* 9(1):22-27.

White, H.E.; Thurston, N.E.; Blackmore, K.A.; Green, S.E.; and Hannah, K.J. 1987. Body temperature in the elderly surgical patient. *Research in Nursing and Health* 10:317-321.

Wirtz, B.J. 1987. Effects of air and water mattresses on thermal regulation. *Journal of Gerontological Nursing* 13(5):13-17.

Table 4.10 / Technical Quality of Care: Exercise

Bassett, C.; McClamrock, E.; and Schmelzer, M. 1982. A 10-week exercise program for senior citizens. *Geriatric Nursing* 3(2):103-105.

Byers, P.H. 1985. Effect of exercise on morning stiffness and mobility in patients with rheumatoid arthritis. *Research in Nursing and Health* 8(3):275-281.

Clough, D. and Maurin, J. 1983. ROM versus NRx. *Journal of Gerontological Nursing* 9(5):278-286.

Colanowski, A. and Gunter, L. 1988. Do retired career women exercise? *Geriatric Nursing* 9(6):350-352.

Gueldner, S. and Spradley, J. 1988. Outdoor walking lowers fatigue. *Journal of Gerontological Nursing* 14(10):6-12.

Karl, C. 1982. The effect of an exercise program on self-care activities for the institutionalized elderly. *Journal of Gerontological Nursing* 8(5):282-285.

Magnani, L.I. 1986. The relationship of hardiness and self-perceived health to activity in groups of independently functioning older adults. *Dissertation Abstracts* 46(12):4184B.

Melillo, K. 1980. Informal activity involvement and the perceived rate of time passage for an older institutionalized population. *Journal of Gerontological Nursing* 6(7):392.

Parent, C. and Wahll, A. 1984. Are physical activity, self-esteem, and depression related? *Journal of Gerontological Nursing* 10(9):8-10.

Roberts, B.L. and Lincoln, R.E. 1988. Cognitive disturbance in hospitalization and institutionalized elderly. *Research in Nursing and Health* 11(5):309-319.

Table 4.11 / Technical Quality of Care: Foot Care

Brown, M.M.; Boosinger, J.; Black, J.; Gaspar, T.; and Sather, L. 1982. Nursing innovation for dry skin care of the feet in the elderly: A demonstration project. *Journal of Gerontological Nursing* 8(7):393-395.

Chung, S. 1983. Foot care: A health care maintenance program. *Journal of Gerontological Nursing* 9(4):212-227.

Frantz, R.A. and Kinney, C.K. 1986. Variables associated with skin dryness in the elderly. *Nursing Research* 35(2):98-100.

Haviland, S. and Garlinghouse, C. 1985. Nursing foot clinics fulfill a great need. *Geriatric Nursing* 6(6):338-341.

Schank, M.J. and Conrad, D. 1977. A survey of the well-elderly and their footproblems, practices, and needs. *Journal of Gerontological Nursing* 3(6):10-15.

Table 4.12 / Technical Quality of Care: Health Teaching Needs

Bahr, S.R. and Griss, L. 1982. Blood pressure readings and selected parameter relationships in an elderly ambulatory population. *Journal of Gerontological Nursing* 8(3):159-163.

Baldini, J. 1981. Knowledge about hypertension in affected elderly persons. *Journal of Gerontological Nursing* 7(9):542-545, 551.

Check, J. and Wurzbach, M. 1984. How elders view learning. *Geriatric Nursing* 5(1):37-39.

Craig, L.L. 1988. Characteristics of older men and their ability to comprehend printed health education materials. *Dissertation Abstracts* 49(4):1088B.

DeBlase, R.; Badziong, M.R.; and Jones, S.L. 1988. Postintraocular lens implants: Needs of patients. *Geriatric Nursing* 9(6):342-343.

Hathaway, D. 1986. Effect of pre-operative instruction on postoperative outcomes: Ameta-analysis. *Nursing Research* 35(5):269-275.

Kim, K.K. 1986. Response time and health care learning of elderly patients. *Research in Nursing and Health* 9(3):233-239.

Lashley, M.E. 1987. Predictors of breast self-examination practice among elderly women. *Advances in Nursing Science* 9(4):25-34.

Shamanasky, S. and Hamilton, W. 1979. The health behavioral awareness test: Self-care education for the elderly. *Journal of Gerontological Nursing* 5(1):29-32.

Table 4.13 / Technical Quality of Care: Confusion

Bernier, S.L. and Small, N.R. 1988. Disruptive behaviors. *Journal of Gerontological Nursing* 14(2):8-13.

Burgio, L.; Jones, L.; and Engel, B. 1988. Studying incontinence in an urban nursing home. *Journal of Gerontological Nursing* 14(4):40-45.

Campbell, E.B.; Williams, M.D.; and Mlynarczyk, S.M. 1986. After the fall: Confusion. *American Journal of Nursing* 86(2):151-154.

Chisholm, S.E.; Denniston, O.L.; Igrisan, R.M.; and Barbus, A.J. 1982. Prevalence of confusion in elderly hospitalized patients. *Journal of Gerontological Nursing* 8(2):87-96.

Clendaniel, B. and Fleishell, A. 1989. An Alzheimer day care center for nursing home patients. *American Journal of Nursing* 89(7):944-945.

Doyle, G.C.; Dunn, S.I.; Thadani, I.; and Lenihan, P. 1986. Investigating tools to aid in restorative care for Alzheimer's patients. *Journal of Gerontological Nursing* 12(9):19-24.

Eaton, M.; Mitchell-Bonair, I.L.; and Friedmann, E. 1986. The effect of touch on nutritional intake of chronic organic brain syndrome patients. *Journal of Gerontology* 41(5):611.

Eisenberg, M.G. and Tierney, D.O. 1985. Profiling disruptive patient incidents. *Quality Review Bulletin* 11(8):245-248.

Evans, L. 1987. Sundown syndrome in institutionalized elderly. *Journal of the American Geriatrics Society* 35(2):101-108.

Foreman, M. 1987. Reliability and validity of mental status questionnaires in elderly hospitalized patients. *Nursing Research* 36(4):217-220.

———.1989. Confusion in the hospitalized elderly: Incidence, onset, and associated factors. *Research in Nursing and Health* 12:21-29.

Hussian, R.A. and Brown, D.C. 1987. Use of two-dimensional grid patterns to limit hazardous ambulation in demented patients. *Journal of Gerontology* 42(5):558-560.

Johnston, L. and Gueldner, S. 1989. Using mnemonics to boost memory in the elderly. *Journal of Gerontological Nursing* 15(8):22-26.

Jones, M. 1985. Patient violence: Report of 200 incidents. *Journal of Psychosocial Nursing* 23(6):12-17.

Langland, R. and Panicucci, C. 1983. Effects of touch on communication with elderly confused clients. *Journal of Gerontological Nursing* 8(3):152-155.

Lincoln, R. 1984. What do nurses know about confusion in the aged? *Journal of Gerontological Nursing* 10(8):26-32.

Maas, M.D. and Buckwalter, K. 1988. A special Alzheimer's unit: Phase I baseline data. *Applied Nursing Research* 1(1):41.

Maddox, M. 1990. Is there a link between dementia and phenylketonuria? *Journal of Gerontological Nursing* 16(5):18-23.

Mayers, K. and Griffin, M. 1990. The play project: Use of stimulus objects with demented patients. *Journal of Gerontological Nursing* 16(1):32-37.

McCracken, A. and Fitzwater, E. 1989. The right environment for Alzheimer's. *Geriatric Nursing* 10(6):293-294.

Nagley, S.J. 1986. Predicting and preventing confusion in your patients. *Journal of Gerontological Nursing* 12(3):27-31.

Negley, E. and Manley, J. 1990. Environmental intervention in assaultive behavior. *Journal of Gerontological Nursing* 16(3):29-33.

Niemoller, J. 1990. Change of pace for Alzheimer's patients. *Geriatric Nursing* 11(2):86-87.

Palmateer, L.M. and McCartney, J.R. 1985. Do nurses know when patients have cognitive deficits? *Journal of Gerontological Nursing* 11(2):6-16.

Richter, J. 1989. Providing nursing home care for the chronically mentally ill. *Journal of Gerontological Nursing* 15(6):18-23.

Roberts, B.L. and Lincoln, R.E. 1988. Cognitive disturbance in hospitalization and institutionalized elderly. *Research in Nursing and Health* 11(5):309-319.

Rosswurm, M. 1989. Assessment of perceptual processing deficits in persons with Alzheimer's disease. *Western Journal of Nursing Research* 11(4):456-468.

Ryden, M. and Knopman, D. 1989. Assess not assume: Measuring the morale of cognitively impaired elderly. *Journal of Gerontological Nursing* 15(11):27-32.

Shomaker, D. 1987. Problematic behavior in the Alzheimer's patient: Retrospection as a method of understanding and counseling. *The Gerontologist* 27(3):370-375.

Struble, L. and Sivertsen, L. 1987. Agitation behaviors in confused elderly patients. *Journal of Gerontological Nursing* 13(11):40-44.

Vermeersch, P.E. 1987. Development of a scale to measure confusion in hospitalized adults. *Dissertation Abstracts* 48:3709B.

Williams, M.; Campbell, E.; Raynor, W.; Mlynarczyk, S.; and Ward, S. 1985. Reducing acute confusional states in elderly patients with hip fractures. *Research in Nursing and Health* 8:329-337.

Williams, M.; Campbell, E.; Raynor, W.; Muscholt, M.; Mlynarczyk, S.; and Crane, L.1985. Predictors of acute confusional states in hospitalized elderly patients. *Research in Nursing and Health* 8:31-40.

Williams, M.; Holloway, J.; Winn, M.; Wolanin, M.; Lawler, M.; Westwick, C.; and Chin, M. 1979. Nursing activities and acute confusional states in elderly hip-fractured patients. *Nursing Research* 28(1):25-35.

Williams, M.; Ward, S.; and Campbell, E. 1988. Confusion: Testing versus observation. *Journal of Gerontological Nursing* 14(1):25-30.

Wiltzius, F.; Gambert, S.; and Duthie, E. 1981. The importance of resident placement within a skilled nursing facility. *Journal of the American Geriatrics Society* 29(9):418-421.

Winger, J. and Schirm, V. 1989. Managing aggressive elderly in long-term care. *Journal of Gerontological Nursing* 15(2):28-33.

Young, S.; Muir-Nash, J.; and Ninos, M. 1988. Managing nocturnal wandering behavior. *Journal of Gerontological Nursing* 4(3):6-12.

Zimmer, J.; Watson, N.; and Treat, A. 1984. Behavioral problems among patients in skilled nursing facilities. *American Journal of Public Health* 74(10):1118-1121.

Table 4.14 / Technical Quality of Care: Bereavement

Constantino, R.E. 1988. Comparison of two group interventions for the bereaved. *Image: The Journal of Nursing Scholarship* 20:83-87.

Farnsworth, J. 1988. The influence of self esteem on the subjective well-being of older divorced and widowed adults. *Dissertation Abstracts* 48(9):2603B.

Gass, K.A. 1987a. Coping strategies of widows. *Journal of Gerontological Nursing* 13(8):29-33.

————.1987b. The health of conjugally bereaved older widows: The role of appraisal, coping, and resources. *Research in Nursing and Health* 19(1):39-47.

————.1988. Aged widows and widowers: Similarities and differences in appraisal, coping, resources, type of death, and health dysfunction. *Archives of Psychiatric Nursing* 2(4):200-210.

Gass, K.A. and Chang, A.S. 1989. Appraisals of bereavement, coping resources, and psychosocial health dysfunction in widows and widowers. *Nursing Research* 38(1):31-36.

Herth, K. 1990. Relationship of hope, coping styles, concurrent losses and setting to grief resolution in the elderly widow(er). *Research in Nursing and Health* 13(2):109-117.

Kirschling, J.M. and Austin, J.K. 1988. Assessing support: The recently widowed. *Archives of Psychiatric Nursing* 2(2):81-86.

Remondet, J. and Hansson, R.O. 1987. Assessing a widow's grief: A short index. *Journal of Gerontological Nursing* 13(4):31-34.

Richter, J. 1989. Providing nursing home care for the chronically mentally ill. *Journal of Gerontological Nursing* 15(6):18-23.

Valanis, B. and Yeaworth, R. 1982. Ratings of physical and mental health in the older bereaved. *Research in Nursing and Health* 5:137-146.

Valanis, B.; Yeaworth, R.; and Mullis, M. 1987. Alcohol use among bereaved and nonbereaved older persons. *Journal of Gerontological Nursing* 13(5):26-32.

Warner, S.L. 1987. A comparative study of widows' and widowers' perceived social support during the first year of bereavement. *Archives of Psychiatric Nursing* 1(4):241-250.

Table 4.15 / Technical Quality of Care: Relocation

Amenta, M.; Weiner, A.; and Amenta, D. 1984. Successful relocation of elderly residents. *Geriatric Nursing* 5(8):356-360.

Bellin, C. 1990. Relocating adult day care: Its impact on persons with dementia. *Journal of Gerontological Nursing* 16(3):11-14.

Brooke, V. 1988. Adjusting to living in a nursing home: Toward a nursing home intervention model. *Dissertation Abstracts* 48(8):2259B.

————.1989. How elders adjust. *Geriatric Nursing* 10(2):66-68.

Chenitz, W. C. 1983. Entry into a nursing home as a status passage: A theory to guide nursing practice. *Geriatric Nursing* 4(2):92-97.

Engle, V. 1985. Temporary relocation: Is it stressful to your patients? *Journal of Gerontological Nursing* 11(10):28-31.

King, F.E.; Figge, J.; and Harman, P. 1986. The elderly coping at home: A study of continuity of nursing care. *Journal of Advanced Nursing* 11:41-46.

McCracken, A. 1987. Emotional impact of possession loss. *Journal of Gerontological Nursing* 13(2):14-19.

Petrou, M. and Obenchain, J. 1987. Reducing incidence of illness post-transfer. *Geriatric Nursing* 8(5):264-266.

Rantz, M. and Egan, K. 1987. Reducing death from translocation syndrome. *American Journal of Nursing* 87(10):1351-1352.

Table 4.16 / Technical Quality of Care: End-of-Life Directives

Bedell, S.E. and Delbanco, T.L. 1984. Choices about cardiopulmonary resuscitation in the hospital: When do physicians talk with patients? *New England Journal of Medicine* 310:1089-1093.

Bedell, S.E.; Pelle, D.; Maher, R.L.; and Cleary, P.D. 1986. Do-not-resuscitate orders for critically ill patients in the hospital: How are they used and what is their impact? *Journal of the American Medical Association* 256(2):233-237.

Cassels, E.J. 1988. Autonomy in the intensive care unit: The refusal of treatment. *Critical Care Clinics*:37.

Jezierski, M. 1988. Minneapolis pre-hospital do-not-resuscitate form. *Journal of Emergency Nursing* 14(4):26-29A.

Justin, R.G. and Johnson, R.A. 1989. Recording end-of-life directives on hospital admission. *Nursing Management* 20(3):65-68.

Lewandowski, W.; Daly, B.; McClish, D.K.; Juknialis, B.W.; and Younger, S.J. 1985. Treatment and care of "do not resuscitate" patients in a medical intensive care unit. *Heart and Lung* 14:175-181.

Shelley, S.I.; Zahorchak, R.M.; and Gambrill, C.D.S. 1987. Aggressiveness of nursing care for older patients and those with do-not-resuscitate orders. *Nursing Research* 36(3):157-162.

Table 4.17 / Technical Quality of Care: Family Caregiver Issues

Baillie, V.; Norbeck, J.S.; and Barnes, L. 1988. Stress, social support, and psychological distress of family care givers of the elderly. *Nursing Research* 37:217-222.

Bowers, B.J. 1987. Intergenerational care giving: Adult care givers and their aging parents. *Advances in Nursing Science* 9(2):20-31.

Bryant, N.H.; Candland, L.; and Lowenstein, R. 1974. Comparison of care and cost outcomes for stroke patients with and without home care. *Stroke* 5:54-59.

Cora, V.L. 1986. Family life process of intergenerational families with functionally dependent elders. *Dissertation Abstracts* 47(3):568B.

Corbin, J.M. and Strauss, A.L. 1984. Collaboration: Couples working together to manage chronic illness. *Image: The Journal of Nursing Scholarship* 16:109-115.

Ethridge, P. and Lamb, G.S. 1989. Professional nursing case management improves quality, access, and costs. *Nursing Management* 20(3):30-35.

Fulmer, T. and Ashley, J. 1989. Clinical indicators of elder neglect. *Applied Nursing Research* 2:161-167.

Gaynor, S. 1989. When the care giver becomes the patient. *Geriatric Nursing* 10(3):120-125.

Given, B.; King, S.; Collins, C.; and Given, C. 1988. Family caregivers of the elderly: Involvement and reactions to care. *Archives of Psychiatric Nursing* 2(5):281-288.

Given, B.; Stommel, M.; Collins, C.; King, S.; and Given, C. 1990. Responses of elderly spouse caregivers. *Research in Nursing and Health* 13(2):77-85.

Graham, R. 1989. Adult day care: How families of dementia patients respond. *Journal of Gerontological Nursing* 15(3):27-31.

Johnson, M. and Maguire, M. 1989. Give me a break: Benefits of a care giver support service. *Journal of Gerontological Nursing* 15(11):22-26.

Kalayjian, A. 1989. Coping with cancer: The spouse's perspective. *Archives of Psychiatric Nursing* 3(3):166-172.

Lund, D.; Feinhauer, L.; and Miller, J. 1985. Living together: Grandparents and children tell their problems. *Journal of Gerontological Nursing* 11(11):29-33.

Phillips, L.R. and Rempusheski, V.F. 1985. A decision-making model for diagnosing and intervening in elder abuse and neglect. *Nursing Research* 34(3):134-139.

————. 1986. Caring for the frail elderly at home: Toward a theoretical explanation of the dynamics of poor quality family care giving. *Advances in Nursing Science* 8(4):62-84.

Robinson, K.M. 1988. A social skills training program for adult caregivers. *Advances in Nursing Science* 10(2):59-72.

————. 1989a. Adjustment to caregiving in older wives: Variations in social support, health, and past marital adjustment. *Dissertation Abstracts* 49(7).

————. 1989b. Predictors of depression among wife caregivers' experience. *Nursing Research* 38(6):359-363.

Sexton, D.L. 1984. The supporting cast: Wives of COPD patients. *Journal of Gerontological Nursing* 10(2):82-85.

Sexton, D.L. and Munro, B.H. 1985. Impact of a husband's chronic illness (COPD) on the spouse's life. *Research in Nursing and Health* 8(1):83-90.

Shomaker, D. 1987. Problematic behavior in the Alzheimer's patient: Retrospection as a method of understanding and counseling. *The Gerontologist* 27(3):370-375.

Wilson, H.S. 1989a. Family caregiving for a relative with Alzheimer's dementia: Coping with negative choices. *Nursing Research* 38:94-98.

———. 1989b. Family caregivers: The experience of Alzheimer's disease. *Applied Nursing Research* 2(1):40-45.

Table 4.18 / Technical Quality of Care: Nursing Home Placement Decision Criteria

Goto, L. and Braun, C. 1987. Nursing home without walls. *Journal of Gerontological Nursing* 13(1):7-9.

Humphreys, D.; Mason, R.; Guthrie, M.; Liem, C.; and Stern, E.J. 1988. The Miami channeling program: Case management and cost control. *Quality Review Bulletin* 14(5):154-160.

Jamieson, M. 1990. Block nursing: Practicing autonomous professional nursing in the community. *Nursing and Health Care* 11(5):250-263.

Jamieson, M.; Campbell, J.; and Clarke, S. 1989. The block nurse program. *The Gerontologist* 29(1):124-127.

Johnson, M. and Werner, C. 1982. We had no choice: A study in familial guilt feelings surrounding nursing home care. *Journal of Gerontological Nursing* 8(11):641-654.

Kaplan, S.W. 1988. An investigation of day care facilities for care of the moderately to severely demented older adults. *Dissertation Abstracts* 49(6):2129B.

Matthiesen, V. 1989. Guilt and grief when daughters place mothers in nursing homes. *Journal of Gerontological Nursing* 15(7):11-15.

McCann, J.J. 1988. Long-term home care for the elderly: Perceptions of nurses, physicians, and primary caregivers. *Quality Review Bulletin* 14(3):66-74.

Mumma, N.L. 1987. Quality and cost control of home care services through coordinated funding. *Quality Review Bulletin* 13(8):271-278.

Schultz, P.R. and Magilvy, J. 1988. Assessing community health needs of the elderly population: Comparisons of three strategies. *Journal of Advanced Nursing* 13:193-202.

Schultz, P.R. and McGlone, F. 1977. Primary health care provided to the elderly by a nurse practitioner/physician team: Analysis of cost-effectiveness. *Journal of the American Geriatrics Society* 25(10):443-446.

Smallegan, M. 1981. Decision making for nursing home admission: A preliminary study. *Journal of Gerontological Nursing* 7(5):280-285.

———. 1985. There was nothing else to do: Needs for care before nursing home admission. *The Gerontologist* 25(4):364-369.

Sullivan, J. and Armignacco, F. 1979. Effectiveness of a comprehensive health program for the well elderly by community health nurses. *Nursing Research* 28(2):70-75.

Worcester, M.H. and Quayhagen, M.P. 1983. Correlates of caregiving satisfaction: Prerequisites to elderly home care. *Research in Nursing Health* 6(2):61-67.

Table 4.19 / Technical Quality of Care: Nursing Staff Issues

Allen, J. 1989. Learning after graduation: Are nurses taking advantage of the resources? *Journal of Gerontological Nursing* 15(8):27-32.

Cambel, S.D. 1985. Primary nursing: It works in long-term care. *Journal of Gerontological Nursing*

Caudill, M. and Patrick, M. 1989. Nursing assistant turnover in nursing homes and need satisfaction. *Journal of Gerontological Nursing* 15(6):24-30.

Chaisson, M.; Beutler, L.; Yost, E.; and Allender, J. 1984. Treating the depressed elderly. *Journal of Psychosocial Nursing* 22 (5):25-30.

Chandler, J.; Rachal, J.; and Kazelskis, R. 1986. Attitudes of long-term care nursing personnel toward the elderly. *The Gerontologist* 26(5): 551-555.

Chisholm, S.E.; Denniston, O.L.; Igrisan, R.M.; and Barbus, A.J. 1982. Prevalence of confusion in elderly hospitalized patients. *Journal of Gerontological Nursing* 8(2):87-96.

Cronin, S.N. and Harrison, B. 1988. Importance of nurse caring behaviors as perceived by patients after myocardial infarction. *Heart and Lung* 17:374-380.

Cuyu, L. and Caltreider, D.L. 1987. Stressed nurses dealing with incontinent patients. *Journal of Gerontological Nursing* 13(1):27-30.

Doering, E.R. 1983. Factors influencing inpatient satisfaction with care. *Quality Review Bulletin* 9(10):291-299.

Ebersole, P. 1985a. *Overcoming the bias of ageism in long-term care.* New York: National League for Nursing.

———. 1985b. Gerontological nurse practitioners, past and present. *Geriatric Nursing* 6(4):219-222.

Glasspoole, L. and Aman, M. 1990. Knowledge, attitudes, and happiness of nurses working with gerontological patients. *Journal of Gerontological Nursing* 16(2):11-14.

Gomez, G.E.; Otto, D.; Blattstein, A.; and Gomez, E.A. 1985. Beginning nursing students can change attitudes about the aged. *Journal of Gerontological Nursing* 11(1):6-11.

Haff, J.; McGowan, C.; Potts, C.; and Streekstra, C. 1988. Evaluating primary nursing in long-term care: Provider and consumer opinions. *Journal of Nursing Quality Assurance* 2(3):44-53.

Harris, M.D. 1988. The changing scene in community health nursing. *Nursing Clinics of North America* 23(3):559-568.

Heater, B.; Becker, A.; and Olson, R. 1988. Nursing interventions and patient outcomes: A meta-analysis of studies. *Nursing Research* 37(5):303-307.

Huss, J.; Buckwalter, K.; and Stolley, J. 1988. Nursing's impact on life satisfaction. *Journal of Gerontological Nursing* 14(5):31-36.

Johnson, J. 1987. Selecting nursing activities for hospitalized clients. *Journal of Gerontological Nursing* 13(10):29-33.

Jones, M. 1985. Patient violence: Report of 200 incidents. *Journal of Psychosocial Nursing* 23(6):12-17.

Knaus, W.A.; Draper, E.A.; Wagner, D.P.; and Zimmerman, J.E. 1986. Evaluation of outcomes from intensive care in major medical centers. *Annals of Internal Medicine* 104:410-418.

Kovner, C.T. 1986. Relationship of nurse-patient agreement on importance of outcomes to patient satisfaction and length of stay. *Dissertation Abstracts* 46:2624B.

Langland, R. and Panicucci, C. 1983. Effects of touch on communication with elderly confused clients. *Journal of Gerontological Nursing* 8(3):152-155.

Lincoln, R. 1984. What do nurses know about confusion in the aged? *Journal of Gerontological Nursing* 10(8):26-32.

Linn, M.W.; Gurel, L.; and Linn, B.S. 1977. Patient outcome as a measure of quality of nursing home care. *American Journal of Public Health* 67(4):337-344.

Loveridge, K. and Heineken, J. 1988. Confirming interactions. *Journal of Gerontological Nursing* 14(5):27-30.

Mech, A.B. 1980. Evaluating the process of nursing care in long-term care facilities. *Quarterly Review Bulletin* 6(3):24-30.

Miller, S.P. and Russel, D. 1980. Elements promoting satisfaction as identified by residents in the nursing home. *Journal of Gerontological Nursing* 6(3):121.

Palmer, M.; McCormick, K.; and Langord, A. 1989. Do nurses consistently document incontinence? *Journal of Gerontological Nursing* 15(12):11-16.

Rosendahl, P. and Ross, V. 1982. Does your behavior affect your patient's response? *Journal of Gerontological Nursing* 8(10):572-575.

Schultz, P.R. and Magilvy, J. 1988. Assessing community health needs of the elderly population: Comparisons of three strategies. *Journal of Advanced Nursing* 13:193-202.

Schultz, P.R. and McGlone, F. 1977. Primary health care provided to the elderly by a nurse practitioner/physician team: Analysis of cost-effectiveness. *Journal of the American Geriatrics Society* 25(10):443-446.

Shelley, S.I.; Zahorchak, R.M.; and Gambrill, C.D.S. 1987. Aggressiveness of nursing care for older patients and those with do-not-resuscitate orders. *Nursing Research* 36(3):157-162.

Steffes, R. and Thralow, J. 1985. Do uniform colors keep patients awake? *Journal of Gerontological Nursing* 11(7):6-9.

Woolferk, C. 1989. What you can expect of nurses aides. *Geriatric Nursing* 10(4):178-180.

Yauger, R.A. 1984. Non-nursing clerical functions: Time, cost, and effect on patient care. *Quality Review Bulletin* 10(2):54-56.

Table 5.1 / Intervention Programs to Improve the Quality of Geriatric Care: Quality Assurance Programs

Bohnet, N.L. 1982. Quality assessment as an ongoing component of hospice care. *Quality Review Bulletin* 8(5):7-20.

Distel, L. 1982. A nursing quality assurance investigation of orthopedic patient care. *Quality Review Bulletin* 8(10):20-22.

Gustafson, D.; Fiss, C.; Frayback, J.; Smelser, P.; and Hiles, M. 1980. Measuring the quality of care in nursing homes: A pilot study in Wisconsin. *Public Health Reports* 95(4):336-343.

Hart, M.A. and Sliefert, M.K. 1983. Monitoring patient incidents in a long-term care facility. *Quality Review Bulletin* 9(12):356-365.

McMillan, B.A. and Jasmund, J.M. 1985. A quality assurance study of height and weight measurement. *Quality Review Bulletin* 11(2):53-56.

Mezey, M.; Lynaugh, J.; and Cherry, J. 1984. The teaching nursing home program. *Nursing Outlook* 32(3):146-150.

Mohide, E.A.; Tugwell, P.; Caulfield, P.; Chambers, L.; Dunnett, C.; Baptiste, S.; Byne, R.; Patterson, C.; Rudnick, V.; and Pill, M. 1988. A randomized trial of quality assurance in nursing homes. *Medical Care* 26(6):554-556.

Neubauer, J.; LeSage, J.; and Roberts, C. 1989. Making the family a partner in quality assurance. *Geriatric Nursing* 10(1):35-37.

Petrucci, C.; McCormick, C.; and Scheve, A. 1987. Documenting patient care needs: Do nurses do it? *Journal of Gerontological Nursing* 13(11):34-38.

Whiteneck, M.R. 1988. Integrating ethics with quality assurance in long-term care. *Quality Review Bulletin* 14(5):138-143.

Table 5.2 / Intervention Programs to Improve the Quality of Geriatric Care: Examples of Quality Assurance Tools

Abrahams, R. and Lamb, S. 1988. Developing reliable assessment in case-managed geriatric long-term care programs. *Quality Review Bulletin* 14(6):179-186.

Hewitt, S.M.; LeSage, J.; Roberts, K.L.; and Ellor, J.R. 1985. Process auditing in long-term care facilities. *Quality Review Bulletin* 11(1):6-16.

Howe, M.; Coulton, M.; Almon, G.; and Sandrick, K. 1980a. Developing scaled outcome criteria for a target patient population. *Quality Review Bulletin 6* (3):17-23.

———. 1980b. Use of scaled outcome criteria for a target patient population. *Quality Review Bulletin* 6(4):15-21.

LaLonde, B. 1987. The general symptom distress scale: A home care outcome measure. *Quality Review Bulletin* 13(7):243-250.

Panniers, T.L. and Newlander, J. 1986. The adverse patient occurrences inventory: Validity, reliability, and implications. *Quality Review Bulletin* 12(9):311-315.

Panniers, T.L. and Tomkiewicz, Z.M. 1985. The ICD-9-CM DRGs: Increased homogeneity through use of AS-SCORE. *Quality Review Bulletin* 11(2):47-52.

Thee, K.G. and Obrecht, W. 1984. Using a patient routing list to document pre-operative instruction. *Quality Review Bulletin* 10(5):149-150.

Ventura, M.R.; Hageman, P.T.; Slakter, M.J.; and Fox, R.N. 1982. Correlations of two quality of nursing care measures. *Research in Nursing and Health* 5(1):32-43.

Table 5.3 / Intervention Programs to Improve the Effectiveness of Health Care

Dinsmore, P. 1979. A health education program for elderly residents in the community. *Nursing Clinics of North America* 14(4):585-593.

Furukawa, C. 1981. Adult health care conference: Community-oriented health maintenance for the elderly. *Journal of Aging and Health Promotion:*105-121.

Goodman, J.J. 1989. Pulmonary rehabilitation and compliance with health care recommendations in chronic bronchitis and emphysema patients. *Dissertation Abstracts* 49(8):3103B.

Harper, D. 1984. Application of Orem's theoretical constructs to self-care medication behaviors in the elderly. *Advances in Nursing Science* 6(3):29-46.

Hilbert, Gail A. 1985. Spouse support and myocardial infarction patient compliance. *Nursing Research* 34(4):217-220.

Jordan-Marsh, M. and Neutra, R. 1985. Relationship of health locus of control and lifestyle change programs. *Research in Nursing and Health* 8(1):3-11.

Kobza, L.L. 1983. Assessing postmastectomy care in a community hospital. *Quality Review Bulletin* 9(4):116-119.

Krommings, S.K. and Ostwald, S.K. 1987. The public health nurse as a discharge planner: Patients' perceptions of the discharge process. *Public Health Nursing* 4:224-229.

Larson, J.L. 1986. Inspiratory muscle training in patients with COPD. *Dissertation Abstracts* 47(1):133B.

Macauley, C.; Murray, L.; and Ellis, H. 1980. Patient-administered drugs in a municipal hospital. *Geriatric Nursing* 1(2):109-111.

McPhee, S.J.; Frank, D.H.; Lewis, C.; Bush, D.E.; and Smith, C.R. 1983. Influence of "discharge interview" on patient knowledge, compliance, and functional status after hospitalization. *Medical Care* 21:755-767.

Naylor, M. 1990. Comprehensive discharge planning for the hospitalized elderly: A pilot study. *Nursing Research* 39(1):42-47.

Pender, N.J. 1985. Effects of progressive muscle relaxation training on anxiety and health locus of control among hypertensive adults. *Research in Nursing and Health* 8(1):67-72.

Perry, J. 1981. Effectiveness of teaching in the rehabilitation of patients with chronic bronchitis and emphysema. *Nursing Research* 30(4):219-228.

Scura, K.W. 1988. Audiological assessment program. *Journal of Gerontological Nursing* 14(10):19-25.

Small, N.R. and Walsh, M.B. 1988. *Teaching nursing homes: The nursing perspective.* Owings Mills, Md.: National Health Publishing.

Stanley, M.J. 1988. Correlates of activity levels for individuals between the ages of 60 and 75 with cardiac disease who have completed a structured cardiac rehabilitation program. *Dissertation Abstracts* 49(6).

Sullivan, J. and Armignacco, F. 1979. Effectiveness of a comprehensive health program for the well elderly by community health nurses. *Nursing Research* 28(2):70-75.

Wilson, R.; Patterson, M.; and Alford, D. 1989. Services for maintaining independence. *Journal of Gerontological Nursing* 15(6):31-37.

Table 5.4 / Intervention Programs to Improve the Quality of Geriatric Care: Examples of Fall Prevention Programs

Campbell, E.B.; Williams, M.D.; and Mlynarczyk, S.M. 1986. After the fall: Confusion. *American Journal of Nursing* 86(2):151-154.

Hendrich, A. 1988. An effective unit-based fall prevention plan. *Journal of Nursing Quality Assurance* 3(1):28-36.

Innes, E.M. 1985. Maintaining fall prevention. *Quality Review Bulletin* 11(7):217-221.

Innes, E.M. and Turman, W.G. 1983. Evaluation of patient falls. *Quality Review Bulletin* 9(2):30-35.

Rainville, N.G. 1984. Effect of an implemented fall prevention program on the frequency of patient falls. *Quality Review Bulletin* 10(9):287-291.

Spellbring, A.; Gannon, M.; Kleckner, T.; and Conway, K. 1988. Improving safety for hospitalized elderly. *Journal of Gerontological Nursing* 14(2):31-37.

Table 5.5 / Intervention Programs to Improve the Quality of Geriatric Care: Risk Factors for Elderly Who Fall

Berryman, E.; Gaskin, D.; Jones, A.; Tolley, F.; and MacMullen G. 1989. Point by point: Predicting elders' falls. *Geriatric Nursing* 10(4):199-201.

Hart, M.A. and Sliefert, M.K. 1983. Monitoring patient incidents in a long-term care facility. *Quality Review Bulletin* 9(12):356-365.

Janken, J.K.; Reynolds, B.A.; and Swiech, K. 1986. Patient falls in the acute caresetting: Identifying risk factors. *Nursing Research* 35(4):215-219.

Johnston, J.E. 1987. Fall prevention responses in the elderly.

   Dissertation Abstracts 48(4):1004B.

———. 1988. The elderly and fall prevention. *Applied Nursing Research* 1(3):140.

Llewellyn, J.; Martin, B.; Shekleton, M.; and Firlit, S. 1988. Analysis of falls in the acute surgical and cardiovascular surgical patient. *Applied Nursing Research* 1(3):116-121.

Morse, J.; Dixon, H.; and Tylko, S. 1985. The patient who falls...and falls again: Defining the aged at risk. *Journal of Gerontological Nursing* 11(11):15-18.

Walshe, A. and Rosen, H. 1979. A study of patient falls from bed. *Journal of Nursing Administration* 9(5):31-35.

Table 5.6 / Intervention Programs to Improve the Mental Status of the Cognitively Impaired Elderly: Reality Orientation, Remotivation, and Resocialization

Citrin, R.S. and Dixon, D.N. 1977. Reality orientation: A milieu therapy used in an institution for the aged. *The Gerontologist* 17(1):39-43.

Cornbleth, T. and Cornbleth, C. 1979. Evaluation of the effectiveness of reality orientation classes in a nursing home unit. *Journal of the American Geriatrics Society* 27(11):522-524.

Gray, P. and Stevenson, J. 1980. Changes in verbal interaction among members of resocialization groups. *Journal of Gerontological Nursing* 6(2):86.

Hanley, I.G. 1981. The use of signposts and active training to modify ward disorientation in elderly patients. *Journal of Behavioral Therapy and Experimental Psychiatry* 12(3):241-247.

Hogstel, M.D. 1979. Use of reality orientation with aging confused patients. *Nursing Research* 28(3):161-165.

Janssen, J. and Giberson, D. 1988. Remotivation therapy. *Journal of Gerontological Nursing* 14(6):31-34.

Mulcahy, N. and Rosa, N. 1981. Reality orientation in a general hospital. *Geriatric Nursing* 2(4):264-268.

Nagley, S.J. 1986. Predicting and preventing confusion in your patients. *Journal of Gerontological Nursing* 12(3):27-31.

Nodhturft, V.L. and Sweeney, N.M. 1982. Reality orientation therapy for the institutionalized elderly. *Journal of Gerontological Nursing* 8(7):396-401.

Reeve, W. and Ivison, D. 1985. Use of environmental manipulation and classroom and modified informal reality orientation with institutionalized, confused elderly patients. *Age and Aging* 14:119-121.

Robb, S.S.; Stegman, C.; and Wolanin, M.O. 1986. No research versus research with compromised results: A study of validation therapy. *Nursing Research* 35(2):113-118.

Settles, H. 1985. A pilot study in reality orientation for the confused elderly. *Journal of Gerontological Nursing* 1(5):11-16.

Tolbert, B.M. 1984. Reality orientation and remotivation in a long-term care facility. *Nursing and Health Care* 5(1):40-44.

Voelkel, D. 1978. A study of reality orientation and resocialization groups with confused elderly. *Journal of Gerontological Nursing* 4(3):13-18.

Zepelin, H.; Wolfe, C.; and Kleinplatz, F. 1981. Evaluation of a year-long reality orientation program. *Journal of Gerontology* 36(1):70-77.

Table 5.7 / Intervention Programs to Improve the Mental Status of the Cognitively Impaired Elderly: Reminiscence

Baker, N. 1985. Reminiscing in group therapy for self-worth. *Journal of Gerontological Nursing* 11(7):21-24.

Hughston, G. and Merriam, S. 1982. Reminiscence: A nonformal technique for improving cognitive functioning in the aged. *International Journal of Aging and Human Development* 15(2):139-149.

Lappe, J.M. 1987. Reminiscing: The life review therapy. *Journal of Gerontological Nursing* 13(4):12-16.

Parsons, W. 1984. Reminiscence group therapy with older persons: A field experiment. *Dissertation Abstracts* 45(4):1040-1041A.

Perrotta, P. and Meacham, J. 1981-82. Can reminiscing intervention alter depression and self-esteem? *International Journal of Aging and Human Development* 14(1):23-30.

Schafer, D. 1985. Reminiscence groups and the institutionalized elderly: An experiment. *Dissertation Abstracts* 46(4):160A.

Walker, L. 1984. The relationships between reminiscing, health state, physical functioning and depression in older adults. *Dissertation Abstracts* 45(5):1432B.

Table 5.8 / Intervention Programs to Improve the Mental Status of the Cognitively Impaired Elderly: Music and Movement Therapy

Goldberg, W. and Fitzpatrick, J. 1980. Movement therapy with the aged. *Nursing Research* 29(6):339-346.

Gueldner, S. and Spradley, J. 1988. Outdoor walking lowers fatigue. *Journal of Gerontological Nursing* 14(10):6-12.

Hartman, L. 1977. The use of music as a program tool with regressed geriatric patients. *Journal of Gerontological Nursing* 3(4):38-42.

Olson, B.K. 1984. Player piano music as therapy for the elderly. *Journal of Music Therapy* 21(1):35-45.

Table 5.9 / Intervention Programs to Improve the Mental Status of the Cognitively Impaired Elderly: Pet Therapy

Andrysco, R. 1982. A study of ethologic and therapeutic factors of pet-facilitated therapy in a retirement nursing community. *Dissertation Abstracts* 43(1):290B.

Baun, M.; Bergstrom, N.; Langston, N.; and Thoma, L. 1984. Physiological effects of human/companion animal bonding. *Nursing Research* 33(3):126-129.

Cowles, K. 1985. The death of a pet: Human responses to the breaking of the bond. *In Pets and the family,* ed. M.B. Sussman, pp. 135-148. New York: HaworthPress.

Francis, G. and Baly, A. 1986. Plush animals: Do they make a difference? *Geriatric Nursing* 7(3):140-142.

Hamilton, G. 1985. The roles of pet and music therapy in providing sensory stimulation to institutionalized elderly persons. *Dissertation Abstracts* 46(4):1059-1060A.

Kongable, L.; Buckwalter, K.; and Stolley, J. 1989. The effects of pet therapy on the social behavior of institutionalized Alzheimer's clients. *Archives of Psychiatric Nursing* 3(4):191-198.

Lauton, M.P.; Moss, M.; and Moles, E. 1984. Pet ownership: A research note. *The Gerontologist* 24(2):208-210.

Lund, D.; Feinhauer, L.; and Miller, J. 1985. Living together: Grandparents and children tell their problems. *Journal of Gerontological Nursing* 11(11):29-33.

Riddick, C.C. 1985. Health, aquariums, and the noninstitutionalized elderly. In *Pets and the family,* ed. M.B. Sussman, pp.163-173. New York: Haworth Press.

Robb, S. and Stegman, C. 1983. Companion animals and elderly people: A challenge for evaluators of social support. *The Gerontologist* 23(3):277-282.

Savishinsky, J. 1985. Pets and family relationships among nursing home residents. In *Pets and the family,* ed. M.B. Sussman, pp. 109-134. New York: Haworth Press.

PROFESSIONAL RESOURCES FOR PROFESSIONAL NURSES
FROM AMERICAN NURSES PUBLISHING!

American Nurses Publishing has the resources for nurses in every kind of setting. Standards of practice, career strategies, legislative information, research — everything that's important to professional nurses.

■ **Standards and Scope of Gerontological Nursing Practice** presents standards for generalists and specialists, with the standards ranging from the organization of nursing services to professional development and ethics. The scope statement focuses on maximizing older persons' self-care abilities. 1987. Pub. No. GE-12. SNA member price $6.50; nonmember price $9.50.

■ **Gerontological Nurses in Clinical Settings: Survey Analysis.** Gives data from the ANA survey on gerontological nurses' education, employment status, experience, nursing activities, satisfaction with work and organization, identification of critical issues, and more. 1986. Pub. No. GE-11. SNA member price $15.50; nonmember price $22.95.

■ **Gerontological Nursing Curriculum: Survey Analysis and Recommendations.** Reports on the ANA study of gerontological nursing curricula in 500 schools; examines such elements as faculty preparation, students' clinical experiences, and the curriculum plan and content. 1986. Pub. No. GE-10. SNA member price $13.50; nonmember price $19.95.

■ **Survival Skills in the Workplace: What Every Nurse Should Know.** This popular new publication provides information on how to make the most of your nursing skills and abilities in today's workplace with its more complex health care services, scarcer financial resources, increasing ethical dilemmas, and personnel shortages. 1990. Pub. No. EC-148. SNA member price $10.75; nonmember price $15.95.

■ **The Nursing Shortage and the 1990s: Realities and Remedies.** How have some institutions overcome shortage problems? Why are nurses leaving nursing? Who's entering nursing and why? This extensive study of nursing shortage in the United States was conducted to answer these and other questions! 1990. Pub. No. G-179. SNA member price $19.95; nonmember price $24.95.

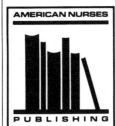

AMERICAN NURSES PUBLISHING

American Nurses Publishing is the publishing program of the American Nurses Association.

TO ORDER ANY OF THESE PUBLICATIONS CALL
(800)637-0323.

FOR A FREE COPY OF THE ANA 1991 PUBLICATIONS CATALOG CALL
(800)274-4ANA.